Pocket Guide for Pharmacy Technicians

■ ■ ■

Jahangir Moini, MD, MPH

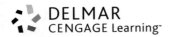

DELMAR
CENGAGE Learning™

**Pocket Guide for
Pharmacy Technicians**
Jahangir Moini

Vice President, Health
Care Business Unit:
William Brottmiller

Editorial Director:
Mathew Kane

Acquisitions Editor:
Kalen Conerly

Senior Product Manager:
Darcy M. Scelsi

Editorial Assistant:
Meaghan O'Brien

Marketing Director:
Jennifer McAvey

Marketing Channel
Manager: Chris Manion

Marketing Coordinator:
Andrea Eobstel

Production Director:
Carolyn Miller

Production Manager:
Barbara A. Bullock

Content Project Manager:
Katie Wachtl

Art Director: Jack Pendleton

© 2008 Delmar, Cengage Learning

For product information and technology assistance,
contact us at **Cengage Learning Customer & Sales
Support, 1-800-354-9706**

For permission to use material from this text
or product, submit all requests online at
www.cengage.com/permissions Further
permissions questions can be emailed to
permissionrequest@cengage.com

Library of Congress Control Number: 2006103500

ISBN-13: 978-1-4180-3221-0

ISBN-10: 1-4180-3221-2

Delmar
Executive Woods
5 Maxwell Drive
Clifton Park, NY 12065
USA

Cengage Learning is a leading provider of customized learning
solutions with office locations around the globe, including Singa-
pore, the United Kingdom, Australia, Mexico, Brazil, and Japan.
Locate your local office at **international.cengage.com/region**

Cengage Learning products are represented in Canada by
Nelson Education, Ltd.

To learn more about Delmar, visit **www.cengage.com/delmar**

Purchase any of our products at your local bookstore or at our
preferred online store **www.ichapters.com**

Printed in the United States of America
4 5 6 7 11 10

■ *This book is dedicated to*

the living memory of my father, and my sister Pari,

my loving and caring family:
mother, wife, and daughters,

and my past and present pharmacy technician
students at Florida Metropolitan University.

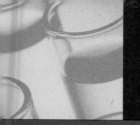

Contents

3 Pharmaceutical Terminology and Abbreviations   25

4 Pharmacy Calculations   49

5 Prescriptions   87

6 Dosage Forms and Administration of Medications   99

7   Community or Retail Pharmacy   119

8 Hospital or Institutional Pharmacy   133

9 Advanced Pharmacy   151

10 Nonsterile Compounding   175

11 Sterile Compounding   209

12 Medication Errors   231

15 Billing and Health Insurance   273

Preface

I believe there is a need for a comprehensive, complete pocket guide for pharmacy technicians that includes not only a quick reference to appropriate procedures, but also includes the duties and responsibilities of a pharmacy technician.

The *Pocket Guide for Pharmacy Technicians* meets these needs both for students and for practicing pharmacy technicians. This reference provides pharmacy technicians all the necessary information related to the knowledge of pharmacology in basic procedural details, pharmacy technician roles and responsibilities, and typical technical considerations.

Chapters 1 through 6 focus on introductions, such as the foundation of pharmaceutical care, drug regulation and control, pharmaceutical terminology, pharmacy calculations, and prescriptions and dosage forms. Chapters 7 through 15 focus on the community and institutional pharmacies and present an overview of these practice settings, financial management, and health insurance. Chapters 16 through 18 focus on drug classification and pharmacologic actions. Appendixes A through O can be used as references to topics such as professional organizations, professional journals, state boards of pharmacy, metric equivalents and conversions, medical symbols and abbreviations, common poisons and their antidotes, common prescribed drugs, controlled substances, pregnancy categories, drug and food interactions, and a full-color visual drug reference.

The book is organized in a natural progression of information: from introductory knowledge to core concepts used daily.

My goal is to empower pharmacy technicians through an understanding of the fundamental skills, duties, and responsibilities in a variety of pharmacy settings.

Dr. Jahangir Moini

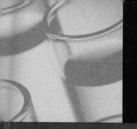

Acknowledgments

I would like to thank:

Darcy Scelsi, for her continual direction and support of this project; Maureen Rosener, who trusted me in my development of this book; Kalen Conerly, Katie Wachtl, and all of the Thomson Delmar Learning staff who have been involved with the creation of this book; the reviewers of this book—whose thorough comments and suggestions were so valuable, and whose insights and eye for detail helped me prepare a more relevant and useful pocket reference; and Greg Vadimsky, who has worked with me side by side since the book's inception.

Also, I would like to thank my wife, Hengi, and my two daughters, who have sacrificed much time away from me while this book was being written.

— Dr. Moini

■ REVIEWERS

Michele Arrowood, CPhT
Certified Pharmacy Technician

James Mizner, RPh, MBA
Pharmacy Technician Program Director
Applied Career Training

Stephanie Mullen, RN, MSN, CPNP
Pediatric Nurse Practitioner
Medical College of Wisconsin

Karen Snipe, CPht, AS, BA, MAEd
Pharmacy Technician Program Coordinator
Trident Technical College

Mary Ann Stuhan, RPh
Pharmacy Program Manager
Cuyahoga Community College

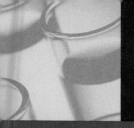

About the Author

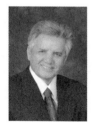

Dr. Moini was assistant professor at Tehran University School of Medicine for nine years teaching medical and allied health students. The author is a professor and former director (for 15 years) of allied health programs at Florida Metropolitan University (FMU). Dr. Moini established, for the first time, the associate degree program for pharmacy technicians in 2000 at FMU's Melbourne campus. For five years, he was the director of the pharmacy technician program. He also established several other new allied health programs for FMU.

Dr. Moini is actively involved in teaching and helping students to prepare for service in various health professions, including the roles of pharmacy technicians, medical assistants, and nurses. He has worked with the Brevard County Health Department as an epidemiologist and health educator consultant since 1990, offering continuing education courses and keeping nurses up to date on the latest developments related to pharmacology, medication errors, immunizations, and other important topics. He has been a published author of various allied health books since 1999.

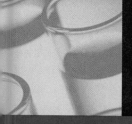

Section I

Introduction

1

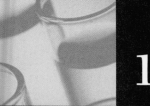

1

The Foundation of Pharmaceutical Care

As the practice of pharmacy evolves, so do the roles of pharmacy technicians. With the rising demand for pharmaceutical products and services, technicians can play a greater role supporting pharmaceutical care. ▪

▪ EDUCATIONAL REQUIREMENTS—PHARMACIST

Most pharmacy colleges now award the *doctor of pharmacy* (Pharm D) degree to students who complete the studies necessary to become pharmacists. This degree requires:

- Two years of pre-pharmacy study, followed by
- Four years of professional studies and experiential rotations

For the BS in Pharm degree, which is increasingly being replaced by the Pharm D degree, the minimum education program, including pre-pharmacy study, is five years.

Specialties in pharmacy may include:

- Ambulatory care
- Pharmacy administration

- Drug information
- Community practice
- Geriatrics
- Industry
- Managed care
- Long-term care
- Home health care
- Oncology
- Nutritional support
- Pediatrics

■ EDUCATIONAL REQUIREMENTS—PHARMACY TECHNICIAN

The core requirements of the two-year associate degree program are the following:

- Administrative and professional aspects of pharmacy
- Terminology
- Calculations (business math and dosage calculations)
- Anatomy
- Pathophysiology
- Pharmacology
- Customer relations
- Health-care delivery systems
- Law and ethics
- Current issues in the practice of pharmacy

- IV admixtures
- Computer applications
- Lab and experiential rotations

CERTIFICATION EXAMINATION FOR THE PHARMACY TECHNICIAN

A **certified pharmacy technician (CPhT)** is a person who has passed the Pharmacy Technician Certification Examination (PTCE) developed and administered by the Pharmacy Technician Certification Board (PTCB). The examination contains questions on the following functional areas:

- Assisting the pharmacist in serving patients—64 percent of the exam
- Maintaining medication and inventory-control systems—25 percent of the exam
- Participating in the administration and management of a pharmacy—11 percent of the exam

  Advantages of certification include:

- Increase in pay
- Promotion in title
- Additional job security
- Expanded job functions and responsibilities
- Increased job satisfaction
- Decreased training time and costs of on-the-job training

■ CONTINUING EDUCATION

In the 1970s, several states acted to require that pharmacists submit evidence of their participation in continuing education as a prerequisite for renewal of their licenses to practice pharmacy. The board of pharmacy in individual states may enact statutes or regulations requiring pharmacists to provide proof of continuing education. The National Association of Boards of Pharmacy (NABP) endorsed mandatory continuing education as a condition for renewal of a license in 1974.

Certification for the pharmacy technician is good for two years and must then be renewed. To become eligible for recertification every 2 years, CPhTs must meet a requirement of 20 contact hours of pharmacy-related continuing education. This can be accomplished through various means, such as:

- Educational meetings
- Seminars
- Workshops
- Conventions

Remember...

Up to 10 contact hours can be earned when the technician is employed under the direct supervision and instruction of a pharmacist.

■ JOB OPPORTUNITIES

Pharmacy technicians with formal training will see increasing job opportunities in all types of pharmacy settings. Employment of pharmacy technicians is expected to grow much faster than the average for all occupations through the year 2010. Reasons for this growth include:

- Numbers of middle-aged and elderly people, who, on average, use more prescription drugs than do younger people, will increase.

- Newer medications will become available to treat more conditions.

- Cost-conscious insurers, pharmacies, and health systems will continue to emphasize the role of pharmacy technicians.

- Pharmacy technicians will continue to assume responsibility for routine tasks previously performed by pharmacists.

- Pharmacy technicians will master new pharmacy technologies, including robotic machinery, so that pharmacy equipment will operate correctly.

■ PLACES OF EMPLOYMENT

The primary employment environments for pharmacists and technicians are:

- Community pharmacies
- Hospitals
- Home care
- Long-term care
- Mail-order pharmacies
- Nuclear pharmacies
- Managed care (insurance companies)

- Pharmaceutical companies
- Ambulatory care centers
- Medical centers
- Teaching facilities
- Outpatient clinics
- Urgent care centers
- Wholesale pharmacies

CODE OF ETHICS

A code of ethics encourages the pharmacist and technician to respect and offer fair treatment for all patients. The following basic principles make up a code of ethics:

- Hold the health and safety of each patient to be of primary consideration.
- Form a professional relationship with each patient.
- Honor the autonomy, values, and dignity of each patient.
- Respect and protect the patient's right of confidentiality.
- Respect the rights of patients to receive pharmacy products and services, and ensure that these rights are met.
- Observe the law, preserve high professional standards, and uphold the dignity and honor of the profession.
- Continuously improve levels of professional knowledge and skills.

- Cooperate with colleagues and other health-care professionals so that maximum benefits to patients are realized.

- Contribute to the health-care system and to the health needs of society.

- Never condone dispensing, promoting, or distributing of drugs or medical devices that do not meet the standards of law or that lack therapeutic value for the patient.

- Be fair and reasonable regarding the amount charged for medications and services.

2

Drug Regulation and Control

Pharmacy technicians must be aware of the legal requirements that apply to their daily professional activities. Laws pertaining to the practice of pharmacy arise from a variety of federal mandates. These mandates are issued from several regulatory agencies in the federal government, including:

- The Food and Drug Administration (FDA)
- The Consumer Product Safety Commission (CPSC)
- The Drug Enforcement Administration (DEA)

State agencies, such as the board of pharmacy, also adopt rules or regulations that in turn become laws. Each state has its own laws pertaining to: the manufacturing, distribution, and dispensing of drugs; requirements of pharmacy technicians; responsibilities and duties of pharmacy technicians; and the pharmacist-to-technician ratio that is required for practice. ∎

FEDERAL FOOD, DRUG, AND COSMETIC ACT (FDCA)

The FDCA was passed in 1938, and its regulations encompass the following:

   a. **Legend drugs**—Legend drugs may be dispensed directly to the patient by means of a valid written or oral prescription from a practitioner, or by a valid refill authorization.

   b. **Over-the-counter (OTC) medications**—OTC medications may be dispensed at retail locations without a prescription. These drugs also may be safely and properly self-administered without the supervision of a physician. OTC preparations must have the following information on the labels:

   - Identity, in boldface, of the OTC product on the principal display panel
   - Adequate directions for use
   - Ingredients in the product
   - Net quantity of the contents
   - Expiration date of the product
   - Lot number of the product
   - Name and place of business of the manufacturer, packager, and/or distributor
   - Disclosure of certain contents and declaration of certain warnings, including pregnancy/nursing warnings, aspirin warnings, and warnings against using acetaminophen for persons who might have compromised liver function

   c. **Generic drugs**—A drug's generic name is usually a short form of the chemical name, a common name, or an official name used in an official compendium.

d. Proprietary drugs—A drug's proprietary name is the name given by the manufacturer to designate the drug's source of manufacture and to differentiate it from the same or chemically similar drugs from other manufacturers. It is also called the **trade name** or **brand name**.

e. Drug recall—Drug recall allows the FDA to initiate regulatory actions to ensure that unsafe, unfit, or ineffective products do not reach the market. Drug recall also allows the FDA to promptly remove those products that do reach the marketplace.

f. Package inserts—The federal government has determined that prescription medication information must be disseminated to health professionals and, in the case of certain drugs, to the patient.

CONTROLLED SUBSTANCES ACT (CSA) OF 1970

This act directs the manufacture, distribution, and dispensing of controlled substances that have the potential for addiction and abuse. This law replaced most previous narcotic and drug abuse laws.

- Certain drugs have a potential for abuse that leads to physical or psychological dependence. As a result, the U.S. government has placed these drugs into schedules (I, II, III, IV, and V) and refers to them as **controlled substances** (see Table 2–1).

- The U.S. attorney general has the authority to add or remove a drug or substance from one of the federal schedules, or to transfer a drug from one federal schedule to another. The federal schedules are updated and published annually by the federal government.

TABLE 2–1   Drug Schedules

Schedule	Description	Examples
I	a. High potential for abuse b. No currently accepted medical use for treatment in the United States c. No acceptable safe use of the drug	Heroin, marijuana, and lysergic acid diethylamide (LSD)
II	a. High potential for abuse b. Currently accepted medical use with severe restrictions c. Abuse of the drug may lead to severe psychological or physical dependence	Amphetamines, cocaine, codeine, hydromorphone, meperidine, methadone, morphine, and opium
III	a. Potential for abuse less than the drugs in Schedules I and II b. Currently accepted medical use in the United States	Acetaminophen with codeine

(continued)

    c. Abuse of the drug may lead to moderate or low physical dependence or high psychological dependence

    d. Some Schedule II drugs are also classified as Schedule III drugs when limited quantities of the Schedule II drug are present in a product

IV   a. Low potential for abuse relative to the drugs in Schedule III   Chloral hydrate, phenobarbital, and benzodiazepines

    b. Currently accepted medical use in the United States

    c. Abuse of the drug may lead to limited physical dependence or psychological dependence relative to the drugs in Schedule III

V   a. Low potential for abuse relative to the drugs in Schedule IV   Lomotil and cough medicines with codeine

(continued)

b. Currently accepted medical use in the United States

c. Abuse of the drug may lead to limited physical dependence or psychological dependence relative to the drugs in Schedule IV

Note: The DEA may place a nonscheduled drug into a scheduled, controlled status after consultation with the FDA. For example, in 1991, certain anabolic steroids were classified as Schedule III drugs because of their abuse potential.

- Schedule I drugs have a high potential for abuse, no currently accepted medical use in the United States, and no acceptable safe use, even under medical supervision.

- Schedule II drugs must be obtained from a supplier (wholesaler or manufacturer) by using **DEA Form 222**. (The CSA does not require the use of any special form to obtain controlled substances in Schedules III–V.)

- All Schedule II controlled substances must be stored in a securely locked, substantially constructed cabinet.

- Every registrant must promptly report any significant loss of Schedule II–V controlled substances to the regional office of the DEA and the Board of Pharmacy. This report must be done using **DEA Form 106**.

- **DEA Form 41** must be submitted to the DEA to dispose of any controlled substance. The DEA will authorize the disposal and instruct the registrant how to dispose of the controlled substance.

  Remember...

  All forms and instructions for completing them can be reviewed, ordered, and downloaded at http://www .deadiversion.usdoj.gov.

POISON PREVENTION PACKAGING ACT (PPPA)

- The PPPA of 1970 requires that drugs for human use in an oral dosage form must be packaged for the consumer in special packaging. Special packaging means **child-resistant containers**—containers designed so that it is significantly difficult and time consuming for children under five years of age to gain access to the packaged medications.

- Special packaging is not required in cases where an OTC medication must be readily available to the elderly or to people with physical challenges. A manufacturer may supply a single size of a drug product in non-child-resistant packaging, as long as it also supplies the medication in packages that use the special packaging. The package must be labeled with the statement: "This package is for households without young children." The package label may also state: "Package not child-resistant."

- The CPSC manages the enforcement functions of the PPPA.

- The following medications are *exempt* from the special packaging requirements:
  - Sublingual dosage forms of nitroglycerin
  - Sublingual and chewable forms of isosorbide dinitrate in dosage strengths of 10 mg or fewer
  - Erythomycin ethylsuccinate granules for oral suspension that do not contain more than 8 grams of equivalent erythromycin
  - Cyclically administered oral contraceptive
  - Anhydrous cholestyramine in powdered form
  - All unit-dose forms of potassium supplements
  - Sodium fluoride drug preparations containing no more than 264 mg of sodium fluoride per package
  - Betamethasone tablets containing no more than 12.6 mg betamethasone
  - Prednisone in tablet form, when containing no more than 105 mg of the drug
  - Mebendazole in tablets containing no more than 600 mg of the drug

■ DRUG LISTING ACT OF 1972

This act assigns a unique and permanent product code, known as a **National Drug Code (NDC)**, to each new drug.

- The NDC identifies the manufacturer, distributor, and formulation, and the size and type of packaging used.
- The FDA maintains a database of drugs by use, manufacturer, and active ingredients, as well as

newly marketed, discontinued, and remarketed drugs by utilizing NDCs.

- Each NDC is unique and cannot be used for another product if any changes occur in product characteristics. A new NDC number must be assigned to any new version of a drug product.

■ DRUG REGULATION REFORM ACT OF 1978

This act eliminated the individual (FDA) approach to regulation and replaced it with a variety of monographs on **drug entities** and **drug product** licenses. It clarified the investigational process used to facilitate and promote research, while protecting patients' rights. It also divided the commercial investigation process into two phases:

1. Drug innovation investigations
2. Drug development investigations

■ OMNIBUS BUDGET RECONCILIATION ACT OF 1990 (OBRA '90)

OBRA '90 mandated that pharmacists perform medication therapy review and provide counseling for individuals (or their caregivers) receiving Medicaid pharmaceutical benefits.

It also provided guidelines for the pharmacist to follow, such as:

- Counseling guidelines
- Documentation requirements
- Extension of standards (applying only to Medicaid patients)

With respect to prescriptions dispensed to Medicaid patients, the federal government has attached certain conditions for reimbursement. As a result, pharmacists are required to do the following in the course of dispensing a Medicaid prescription:

1. Obtain and maintain a history of the patient (a medication history).

2. Conduct a review of every prescription and screen for potential drug therapy/interaction problems.

3. Make an offer to counsel each Medicaid recipient concerning the drug.

OBRA '90 requires manufacturers that want to participate in the Medicaid program to offer the federal government their best (the lowest) price for prescription drugs.

■ OCCUPATIONAL SAFETY AND HEALTH ACT OF 1970

In 1970, Congress passed the Occupational Safety and Health Act. This act established the **Occupational Safety and Health Administration (OSHA)**, charged with writing and enforcing compulsory standards for health and safety in the workplace. The act included regulations for the following:

• Physical workplace
• Machinery and equipment
• Materials
• Power sources

- Processing
- Protective clothing
- First aid
- Administrative requirements

All employers must understand the standards that apply to their business. Many states have employee **right-to-know laws**, which allow employees access to information about the following:

- Toxic or hazardous substances
- Employer duties
- Employee rights
- Other health and safety issues

Hazard Communication Standard (HCS) is an OSHA standard intended to increase health-care practitioners' awareness of risks, improve work practices and appropriate use of personal protective equipment, and reduce injuries and illnesses in the workplace.

■ HEALTH INSURANCE PORTABILITY AND ACCOUNTABILITY ACT (HIPAA '96)

In 1996, the **Health Insurance Portability and Accountability Act (HIPAA)** was signed into law to set a national standard for electronic transfer of health data. Most health-care entities were required to meet the standards set in the privacy issues section of HIPAA on April 14, 2003. HIPAA is federal legislation that requires all health-care providers, including pharmacies, to protect patient information from unauthorized use and disclosure. It is referred to as the

Privacy Rule and was established when the government recognized that individually identifiable health information is readily available due to health-care plans, health-care clearinghouses, third-party billing practices, clinical research trials, and the transmission of health information in electronic form.

Pharmacy technicians work with a significant amount of confidential personal patient information. This information may include:

- Patients' financial records
- Medical records
- Other confidential information

Any discussions of the patient's confidential information can be conducted only with the pharmacist and only within the scope of pharmacy practice.

Protected health information (PHI) must be confidentially maintained by a health-care provider to prevent any unauthorized use or disclosure.

PENALTIES FOR VIOLATION OF THE PRIVACY RULE

Any person who violates the Privacy Rule may not be fined more than $100 for each violation up to a total of $25,000 per calendar year for all violations of an identical requirement. Additional penalties may be imposed for the following *wrongful disclosure* of individually identifiable health information:

- Wrongful disclosure of PHI under false pretenses: fine of not more than $50,000; imprisonment of not more than one year; or both
- Wrongful disclosure of PHI committed with intent to sell, transfer, or use same for commercial

advantage, personal gain, or malicious harm: fine of not more than $250,000; imprisonment of not more than 10 years; or both

■ NEW DRUG APPROVAL

The U.S. FDA regulates all drug products on the market in the United States. It was founded to protect the consumer by ensuring the following:

- Purity
- Potency
- Efficacy
- Safety of drug and food products

■ LAW AND THE PHARMACY TECHNICIAN

Pharmacy technicians should request a copy of the state laws from their State Board of Pharmacy to ensure that their practice of pharmacy is legal and valid. The supervising pharmacist is liable for all actions of pharmacy technicians. As a pharmacy technician, you are obligated to responsibly follow all state and federal laws to the best of your ability. Because you are working under your pharmacist's license, you may be subject to civil judgments, but may not be subject to legal action.

3

Pharmaceutical Terminology and Abbreviations

Medical terminology is the language of medicine used in all areas of the health-care industry. The ability to understand and define the parts of medical terminology will make it easier to understand all medical words, therefore enhancing your ability to communicate precisely with other health-care professionals. Pharmaceutical terminology and abbreviations help the pharmacy technician understand the language of medicine and to dispense prescriptions and medication orders without error. An understanding of pharmaceutical terminology and abbreviations is a must for the pharmacy technician. ■

■ MEDICAL AND PHARMACY ABBREVIATIONS

A list of commonly used abbreviations is shown in Table 3–1. It is important to become familiar with the approved list of abbreviations provided at the facility at which you are working.

TABLE 3–1 Abbreviations Commonly Used in Prescriptions and Medication Orders

Abbreviation	Meaning
aa, $\overline{aa}$	Of each
a.c.	Before meals
ad lib.	At pleasure, as desired
Admin.	Administer
a.m.	Morning
amp.	Ampule
Aq.	Water
ASA	Aspirin
ATC	Around the clock
b.i.d.	Twice a day
BMD	Bone mineral density
BM	Bowel movement
BP	Blood pressure
BS	Blood sugar
BSA	Body surface area
c. or $\overline{c}$	With
cap.	Capsule
CHD	Coronary heart disease
CHF	Congestive heart failure
Comp.	Compound

(continued)

d.	Day
dil.	Dilute
disp.	Dispense
div.	Divide
d.t.d.	Give of such doses
DW	Distilled water
D5LR	Dextrose 5% in lactated Ringer's
D5NS	Dextrose 5% in normal saline (0.9% sodium chloride)
D5W	Dextrose 5% in water
D10W	Dextrose 10% in water
elix.	Elixir
e.o.d.	Every other day
et	And
ex aq.	In water
f. or fl.	Fluid
ft	Make
g	Gram
GI	Gastrointestinal
gl. aq.	Glass of water
GFR	Glomerular filtration rate
gtt.	Drop
GU	Genitourinary
h. or hr.	Hour

(continued)

HA	Headache
HBP	High blood pressure
HC	Hydrocortisone
HRT	Hormone replacement therapy
HT or HTN	Hypertension
ID	Intradermal
IM	Intramuscular
iso.	Isotonic
IV	Intravenous
IVP	Intravenous push
IVPB	Intravenous piggyback
m & n	Morning and night
M.	Mix
min.	Minute
m^2 or M^2	Square meter
mcg	Microgram
mEq	Milliequivalent
mg	Milligram
mg/kg	Milligram (of drug) per kilogram (of body weight)
mg/m^2	Milligram (of drug) per square meter (of body surface area)
MI	Myocardial infarction
mL	Milliliter

(continued)

mL/h	Milliliter (of drug administered) per hour (as through intravenous administration)
N & V	Nausea and vomiting
NF	National Formulary
NMT	Not more than
No.	Number
noct.	Night
non rep. or N.R.	Do not repeat
NPO	Nothing by mouth
N.S. or NS	Normal saline
$\frac{1}{2}$ NS	Half-strength normal saline
NTG	Nitroglycerin
o.l.	Left eye
oint.	Ointment
p.c.	After meals
p.m.	Afternoon; evening
p.o.	By mouth
postop	Postoperatively
ppb	Parts per billion
ppm	Parts per million
p.r.n. or prn	As required
pt.	Patient
pulv.	Powder

(continued)

q.	Every
q.h.	Every hour
q.i.d.	Four times a day
q.s. or qs.	A sufficient quantity
q.s. ad	A sufficient quantity to make
rect.	Rectal or rectum
rep.	Repeat
R.L. or R/L	Ringer's Lactate
Rx	Prescription symbol (recipe, you take)
s. or s̄	Without
s.i.d.	Once a day
Sig.	Write on label
SL	Sublingual
SOB	Shortness of breath
sol.	Solution
s.o.s.	If there is need; as needed
Stat.	Immediately
sup. or supp.	Suppository
susp.	Suspension
syr.	Syrup
tab.	Tablet
t.a.t.	Until all taken
tbsp.	Tablespoonful
t.i.d.	Three times a day

(continued)

top.	Topically
TPN	Total parenteral nutrition
tsp.	Teaspoonful
u.d. or ut. dict.	As directed
ung.	Ointment
URI	Upper respiratory infection
USP	United States Pharmacopoeia
UTI	Urinary tract infection
vol.	Volume
w.a.	While awake
wk.	Week

MEDICATION ERRORS

Medication errors can result from the misuse, misinterpretation, and illegible writing of abbreviations, and through the use of made-up abbreviations. The use of a controlled vocabulary, a reduction in the use of abbreviations, care in the writing of decimal points, and the proper use of leading and terminal zeros have been urged to help reduce medication errors. The Joint Commission has created a Do Not Use list for abbreviations that are prone to cause medication errors (Table 3–2). Further, the Institute for Safe Medication Practices (ISMP) has created a list of Error-Prone abbreviations based on the USP-ISMP Medication Error Reporting Program (Table 3–3).

TABLE 3–2   Official "Do Not Use" List[1]

Do Not Use	Potential Problem	Use Instead
U (unit)	Mistaken for "0" (zero), the number "4" (four) or "cc"	Write "unit"
IU (International Unit)	Mistaken for IV (intravenous) or the number 10 (ten)	Write "International Unit"
Q.D., QD, q.d., qd (daily) Q.O.D., QOD, q.o.d, qod (every other day)	Mistaken for each other Period after the Q mistaken for "I" and the "O" mistaken for "I"	Write "daily" Write "every other day"
Trailing zero (X.0 mg)* Lack of leading zero (.X mg)	Decimal point is missed	Write X mg Write 0.X mg
MS	Can mean morphine sulfate or magnesium sulfate	Write "morphine sulfate" Write "magnesium sulfate"
MSO_4 and $MgSO_4$	Confused for one another	

(continued)

[1] Applies to all orders and all medication-related documentation that is handwritten (including free-text computer entry) or on pre-printed forms.

*Exception: A "trailing zero" may be used only where required to demonstrate the level of precision of the value being reported, such as for laboratory results, imaging studies that report size of lesions, or catheter/tube sizes. It may not be used in medication orders or other medication-related documentation.

Additional Abbreviations, Acronyms and Symbols
(For possible future inclusion in the Official "Do Not Use" List)

Do Not Use	Potential Problem	Use Instead
> (greater than) < (less than)	Misinterpreted as the number "7" (seven) or the letter "L" Confused for one another	Write "greater than" Write "less than"
Abbreviations for drug names	Misinterpreted due to similar abbreviations for multiple drugs	Write drug names in full
Apothecary units	Unfamiliar to many practitioners Confused with metric units	Use metric units

(continued)

@	Mistaken for the number "2" (two)	Write "at"
cc	Mistaken for U (units) when poorly written	Write "ml" or "milliliters"
µg	Mistaken for mg (milligrams) resulting in one thousand-fold overdose	Write "mcg" or "micrograms"

© The Joint Commission. Reprinted with Permission.

ISMP'S LIST OF *ERROR-PRONE ABBREVIATIONS, SYMBOLS,* AND *DOSE DESIGNATIONS*

The abbreviations, symbols, and dose designations found in this table have been reported to ISMP through the USP-ISMP Medication Error Reporting Program as being frequently misinterpreted and involved in harmful medication errors. They should NEVER be used when communicating medical information. This includes internal communications, telephone/verbal prescriptions, computer-generated labels, labels for drug storage bins, medication administration records, as well as pharmacy and prescriber computer order entry screens. The Joint Commission has established a National Patient Safety Goal that specifies that certain abbreviations must appear on an accredited organization's do-not-use list; we have highlighted these items with a double asterisk (**). However, we hope that you will consider others beyond the minimum Joint Commission requirements. By using and promoting safe practices and by educating one another about hazards, we can better protect our patients.

TABLE 3–3 ISMP's List of *Error-Prone Abbreviations, Symbols, and Dose Designations*

Abbreviations	Intended Meaning	Misinterpretation	Correction
μg	Microgram	Mistaken as "mg"	Use "mcg"
AD, AS, AU	Right ear, left ear, each ear	Mistaken as OD, OS, OU (right eye, left eye, each eye)	Use "right ear," "left ear," or "each ear"
OD, OS, OU	Right eye, left eye, each eye	Mistaken as AD, AS, AU (right ear, left ear, each ear)	Use "right eye," "left eye," or "each eye"
BT	Bedtime	Mistaken as "BID" (twice daily)	Use "bedtime"
cc	Cubic centimeters	Mistaken as "u" (units)	Use "mL"
D/C	Discharge or discontinue	Premature discontinuation of medications if D/C (intended to mean "discharge") has been misinterpreted as "discontinued" when followed by a list of discharge medications	Use "discharge" and "discontinue"

(continued)

IJ	Injection	Mistaken as "IV" or "intrajugular"	Use "injection"
IN	Intranasal	Mistaken as "IM" or "IV"	Use "intranasal" or "NAS"
HS	Half-strength	Mistaken as bedtime	Use "half-strength" or "bedtime"
hs	At bedtime, hours of sleep	Mistaken as half-strength	
IU**	International unit	Mistaken as IV (intravenous) or 10 (ten)	Use "units"
o.d. or OD	Once daily	Mistaken as "right eye" (OD-oculus dexter), leading to oral liquid medications administered in the eye	Use "daily"
OJ	Orange juice	Mistaken as OD or OS (right or left eye); drugs meant to be diluted in orange juice may be given in the eye	Use "orange juice"
Per os	By mouth, orally	The "os" can be mistaken as "left eye" (OS-oculus sinister)	Use "PO," "by mouth," or "orally"

(continued)

q.d. or QD**	Every day	Mistaken as q.i.d., especially if the period after the "q" or the tail of the "q" is misunderstood as an "i"	Use "daily"
qhs	Nightly at bedtime	Mistaken as "qhr" or every hour	Use "nightly"
qn	Nightly or at bedtime	Mistaken as "qh" (every hour)	Use "nightly" or "at bedtime"
q.o.d. or QOD**	Every other day	Mistaken as "q.d." (daily) or "q.i.d." (four times daily) if the "o" is poorly written	Use "every other day"
q1d	Daily	Mistaken as q.i.d. (four times daily)	Use "daily"
q6PM, etc.	Every evening at 6 PM	Mistaken as every 6 hours	Use "6 PM nightly" or "6 PM daily"
SC, SQ, sub q	Subcutaneous	SC mistaken as SL (sublingual); SQ mistaken as "5 every"; the "q" in "sub q" has been mistaken as "every" (e.g., a	Use "subcut" or "subcutaneously"

(continued)

	heparin dose ordered "sub q 2 hours before surgery" misunderstood as every 2 hours before surgery)	
ss	Sliding scale (insulin) or $\frac{1}{2}$ (apothecary)	Mistaken as "55"	Spell out "sliding scale;" use "one-half" or "$\frac{1}{2}$"
SSRI	Sliding scale regular insulin	Mistaken as selective-serotonin reuptake inhibitor	Spell out "sliding scale (insulin)"
SSI	Sliding scale insulin	Mistaken as Strong Solution of Iodine (Lugol's)	
i/d	One daily	Mistaken as "tid"	Use "1 daily"
TIW or tiw	3 times a week	Mistaken as "3 times a day" or "twice in a week"	Use "3 times weekly"
U or u**	Unit	Mistaken as the number 0 or 4, causing a 10-fold overdose or greater (e.g., 4U	Use "unit"

(continued)

Dose Designations and Other Information	Intended Meaning	Misinterpretation	Correction
		seen as "40" or 4u seen as "44"); mistaken as "cc" so dose given in volume instead of units (e.g, 4u seen as 4cc)	
Trailing zero after decimal point (e.g., 1.0 mg)**	1 mg	Mistaken as 10 mg if the decimal point is not seen	Do not use trailing zeros for doses expressed in whole numbers
No leading zero before a decimal dose (e.g., .5 mg)**	0.5 mg	Mistaken as 5 mg if the decimal point is not seen	Use zero before a decimal point when the dose is less than a whole unit
Drug name and dose run together (especially	Inderal 40 mg	Mistaken as Inderal 140 mg	Place adequate space between the drug

(continued)

problematic for drug names that end in "l" such as Inderal40 mg; Tegretol300 mg)	Tegretol 300 mg	Mistaken as Tegretol 1300 mg	name, dose, and unit of measure
Numerical dose and unit of measure run together (e.g., 10mg, 100mL)	10 mg 100 mL	The "m" is sometimes mistaken as a zero or two zeros, risking a 10- to 100-fold overdose	Place adequate space between the dose and unit of measure
Abbreviations such as mg or mL with a period following the abbreviation	mg mL	The period is unnecessary and could be mistaken as the number 1 if written poorly	Use mg, mL, etc. without a terminal period
Large doses without properly placed commas (e.g., 100000 units; 1000000 units)	100,000 units 1,000,000 units	100000 has been mistaken as 10,000 or 1,000,000; 1000000 has been mistaken as 100,000	Use commas for dosing units at or above 1,000, or use words such as 100 "thousand" or 1 "million" to improve readability

(continued)

Drug Name Abbreviations	Intended Meaning	Misinterpretation	Correction
ARA A	Vidarabine	Mistaken as cytarabine (ARA C)	Use complete drug name
AZT	Zidovudine (Retrovir)	Mistaken as azathioprine or aztreonam	Use complete drug name
CPZ	Compazine (prochlorperazine)	Mistaken as chlorpromazine	Use complete drug name
DPT	Demerol-Phenergan-Thorazine	Mistaken as diphtheria-pertussis-tetanus (vaccine)	Use complete drug name
DTO	Diluted tincture of opium, or deodorized tincture of opium (Paregoric)	Mistaken as tincture of opium	Use complete drug name

(continued)

HCl	Hydrochloric acid or hydrochloride	Mistaken as potassium chloride (The "H" is misinterpreted as "K")	Use complete drug name unless expressed as a salt of a drug
HCT	Hydrocortisone	Mistaken as hydrochlorothiazide	Use complete drug name
HCTZ	Hydrochlorothiazide (seen as HCT250 mg)	Mistaken as hydrocortisone	Use complete drug name
MgSO4**	Magnesium sulfate	Mistaken as morphine sulfate	Use complete drug name
MS, MSO4**	Morphine sulfate	Mistaken as magnesium sulfate	Use complete drug name
MTX	Methotrexate	Mistaken as mitoxantrone	Use complete drug name
PCA	Procainamide	Mistaken as patient controlled analgesia	Use complete drug name
PTU	Propylthiouracil	Mistaken as mercaptopurine	Use complete drug name
T3	Tylenol with codeine No. 3	Mistaken as liothyronine	Use complete drug name

(continued)

	Intended Meaning	Misinterpretation	Correction
TAC	Triamcinolone	Mistaken as tetracaine, Adrenalin, cocaine	Use complete drug name
TNK	TNKase	Mistaken as "TPA"	Use complete drug name
ZnSO4	Zinc sulfate	Mistaken as morphine sulfate	Use complete drug name
Stemmed Drug Names			
"Nitro" drip	Nitroglycerin infusion	Mistaken as sodium nitroprusside infusion	Use complete drug name
"Norflox"	Norfloxacin	Mistaken as Norflex	Use complete drug name
"IV Vanc"	Intravenous vancomycin	Mistaken as Invanz	Use complete drug name

(continued)

Symbols	Intended Meaning	Misinterpretation	Correction
ʒ	Dram	Symbol for dram mistaken as "3"	Use the metric system
♏	Minim	Symbol for minim mistaken as "mL"	
x3d	For three days	Mistaken as "3 doses"	Use "for three days"
> and <	Greater than and less than	Mistaken as opposite of intended; mistakenly use incorrect symbol; " < 10" mistaken as "40"	Use "greater than" or "less than"
/ (slash mark)	Separates two doses or indicates "per"	Mistaken as the number 1 (e.g., "25 units/10 units" misread as "25 units and 110" units)	Use "per" rather than a slash mark to separate doses
@	At	Mistaken as "2"	Use "at"

(continued)

&	And	Mistaken as "2"	Use "and"
+	Plus or and	Mistaken as "4"	Use "and"
°	Hour	Mistaken as a zero (e.g., q2° seen as q 20)	Use "hr," "h," or "hour"

**These abbreviations are included on The Joint Commission's "minimum list" of dangerous abbreviations, acronyms and symbols that must be included on an organization's "Do Not Use" list, effective January 1, 2004. Visit http://www.jcaho.org for more information about this Joint Commission requirement.

Permission is granted to reproduce material for internal newsletters or communications with proper attribution. Other reproduction is prohibited without written permission. Unless noted, reports were received through the USP-ISMP Medication Errors Reporting Program (MERP). Report actual and potential medication errors to the MERP via the web at http://www.ismp.org or by calling 1-800-FAIL-SAF(E). ISMP guarantees confidentiality of information received and respects reporters' wishes as to the level of detail included in publications.

© ISMP

ARABIC AND ROMAN NUMERALS ON PRESCRIPTIONS

A prescription also may contain a mixture of Arabic and Roman numerals. The Roman system of notation is used to express a large range of numbers by the use of eight base letters of the alphabet in simple "positional" notation to indicate adding to or subtracting from the succession of letter values (Table 3–4).

TABLE 3–4	**Roman Numerals Used in Prescriptions**
Base Letters	Values
SS or ss	$\frac{1}{2}$
I or i	1
V or v	5
X or x	10
L or l	50
C or c	100
D or d	500
M or m	1,000

■ DRUG NAMES

Throughout the development process, drugs may have several names assigned to them: a chemical name, a generic (nonproprietary) name, an official name, and a trade or brand name. This naming convention is confusing unless the pharmacy technician has a clear understanding of the different names used.

- **Generic name**—The most commonly used name. This is the name the manufacturer uses for a drug, and it is the same in all countries.

- **Trade or brand name**—This name is followed by the symbol ®, which indicates that the name is registered to a specific manufacturer or owner, and that no one else can use it.

- **Chemical name**—This name is derived from the drug's chemical composition. This name may be hyphenated and is usually long.

The most commonly used trade names of medications and their corresponding generic names are seen in Appendix G.

4

Pharmacy Calculations

B asic math skills are essential for pharmacy technicians to calculate most dosage and solution problems encountered today in clinical practice. The technician should be familiar with Roman numerals, the different measurement systems, fractions, decimals, and percentages, as well as have the ability to solve for the value of an unknown (X) by using ratio-proportion. ■

■ ARABIC NUMBERS AND ROMAN NUMERALS

- Most medication dosages are prescribed by the physician or another practitioner using the metric and household systems for weights and measures, and by utilizing the Arabic number system and its symbols called **digits or integers** (such as 1, 2, 3, 4, 5, 6, 7, 8, 9, 10).

- Occasionally orders are received in the apothecary system of weights and measures utilizing the Roman numeral system with numbers represented by **symbols** such as I, V, and X. The Roman numeral system uses seven basic symbols and various combinations of these symbols to represent all numbers in the Arabic number system (see Table 4–1). Roman numerals can be written as uppercase or lowercase letters.

TABLE 4–1	**Seven Basic Roman Numerals**
Roman Numerals	Arabic Numbers
I	1
V	5
X	10
L	50
C	100
D	500
M	1000

RULES FOR USING ROMAN NUMERALS

1. No symbol may be used more than three times. The exception is the symbol for five (V), which is used only once because there is a symbol for 10 (X), and a combination of symbols for 15 (XV).

Example:

$$II = (1 + 1) = 2$$
$$XXV = (10 + 10 + 5) = 25$$

2. When symbols of lesser value follow symbols of greater value, they are **added** to construct a number.

Example:

VII $= (5 + 1 + 1)$ $= 7$
XVIII $= (10 + 5 + 1 + 1 + 1)$ $= 18$

3. When symbols of greater value follow symbols of lesser value, those of lesser value are **subtracted** from those of higher value to construct a number.

Example:

IV $= (5 - 1)$ $= 4$
IX $= (10 - 1)$ $= 9$

For examples of Roman numeral equivalents for Arabic numbers, see Table 4–2.

TABLE 4–2	Roman Numeral Equivalents for Arabic Numbers
Arabic Numbers	**Roman Numerals**
$\dfrac{1}{2}$	$\overline{ss}$
1	i
2	ii
3	iii
4	iv
5	v
6	vi
7	vii
8	viii

(continued)

9	ix
10	x
15	xv
20	xx
30	xxx
50	L
100	C
500	D
1000	M

THE METRIC SYSTEM

The metric system is:

- The most accurate and popular system used today for drug prescription and administration
- A decimal system of weights and measures
- Often denoted as **SI** units from the **Système International**

BASIC UNITS OF THE METRIC SYSTEM

The metric system has three basic units of measurement:

- The meter (m) is the unit of length.
- The gram (g) is the unit of weight.
- The liter (L) is the unit of volume.

Weight Equivalents

1 kilogram (kg)	= 1000 grams (g)
1 g	= 1000 milligrams (mg)
	= 1,000,000 micrograms (mcg)

1 mg $= \dfrac{1}{1000}$ g or 0.001 g

or 1000 mcg

1 mcg $= \dfrac{1}{1000}$ mg or 0.001 mg

or 0.000001 g

Volume Equivalents

1 liter (L) = 1000 milliliters (mL)

1 mL $= \dfrac{1}{1000}$ L or 0.001 L

Note: Prescriptions should be fully written out without the use of abbreviations.

THE HOUSEHOLD SYSTEM

- Household measure in the United States is also called *Customary Measurement,* and it is the least accurate measurement system.

- Household measurements are calculated by using containers easily found in the home. Because containers differ in design, size, and capacity, it is impossible to establish a standard unit of measure. Table 4–3 lists common household measurements.

- The instruments used for measurement in this system include medicine droppers, teaspoons, tablespoons, cups, and glasses.

- Pharmacy technicians must be knowledgeable about this system to provide good home health-care services.

TABLE 4–3   Common Household Measurements

Unit	Volume	Symbol
Drop	——	gtt
Teaspoon	60 drops	t or tsp
Tablespoon	3 teaspoons	T or tbsp
Ounce	2 tablespoons	oz
Cup (teacup)	6 ounces	c
Glass or cup	8 ounces	gl
Pint	16 ounces	pt
Quart	2 pints	qt

THE APOTHECARY SYSTEM

- This system of measurement is rare in the clinical setting, and it is one of the oldest of the measurement systems.
- Its basic measure for weight is the grain (gr).
- The apothecary system uses fractions, Roman numerals, and Arabic numbers.

APOTHECARY EQUIVALENTS

1 minim (min)	= 0.06 mL	= 1 gtt
1 dram (dr, ℥)	= approximately 5 mL	= 60 gtt
	= 1 t	
1 ounce (oz or ℥)	= approximately 30 mL	= 2 T
1 pint (pt)	= 16 oz	
1 quart (qt)	= 32 oz	

Table 4–4 shows equivalent measures between the metric, apothecary, and household systems.

TABLE 4–4   Equivalent Measures

Metric		Household		Apothecary
1 mL	=	15 gtt	=	15 min
15 mL	=	1 T	=	4 dr
30 mL	=	1 oz	=	1 oz
473 mL	=	1 pt	=	1 pt
946 mL	=	1 qt	=	1 qt
3785 mL	=	1 gallon	=	1 gallon

INTERNATIONAL UNITS

- An International Unit is defined as the amount of a drug that produces a specific, measurable response in an animal.

- International units are often used to designate the strength of a product when the mass (milligrams, grams, etc.) of the product produces an unreliable clinical effect. For example, drugs such as insulin, heparin, and vitamin E are often measured using standardized tests of their biologic activity (by their units of activity rather than their milligram strength) because the potency of a milligram of each of these drugs varies depending on the animal or plant source from which the drug was derived.

FRACTIONS

- A fraction is a part or piece of a whole that indicates division of that whole into equal units or parts. A fraction is written with one number over another. Figure 4–1 shows examples of parts of a fraction.

- The denominator refers to the total number of pieces and is the number on the bottom of the fraction.

- The numerator refers to the part of the whole that is being considered. This number is on the top of the fraction.

$$\text{Fraction} = \frac{\text{numerator}}{\text{denominator}}$$

- The number on the top of the line (numerator) is divided by the number under the line (denominator).

- Pharmacy technicians need to know how to calculate dosage problems with fractions because fractions are used in apothecary and household measures.

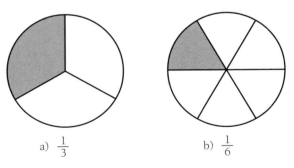

a) $\frac{1}{3}$ b) $\frac{1}{6}$

Example:

FIGURE 4–1 **(a) Three equal parts, or** $\frac{1}{3}$ **per part; and (b) six equal parts, or** $\frac{1}{6}$ **per part.**

TYPES OF FRACTIONS

Common fractions can be divided into four groups:

- Proper fractions
- Improper fractions
- Mixed numbers
- Complex fractions

Proper Fractions

If the numerator is less than the denominator, the fraction value is less than one. These fractions are called **proper fractions**.

Examples:

$$\frac{1}{2} < 1, \frac{3}{5} < 1, \frac{7}{10} < 1$$

Improper Fractions

If the numerator and denominator are equal to each other, the fraction's value is equal to one. These fractions are called **improper fractions**.

Examples:

$$\frac{4}{4} = 1, \frac{9}{9} = 1, \frac{16}{16} = 1$$

If the numerator is greater than the denominator, the fraction's value is greater than one. These fractions are also called **improper fractions**.

Examples:

$$\frac{4}{3} = 4 > 3 \quad \frac{7}{5} = 7 > 5$$

Mixed Numbers

If a fraction and a whole number are written together, the fraction's value is always greater than one. These fractions are called **mixed numbers**.

Examples:

$$1\frac{1}{2} > 1, \ 2\frac{2}{3} > 1, \ 7\frac{3}{4} > 1$$

Complex Fractions

If a fraction has a combination of whole numbers and proper and improper fractions in both the numerator and the denominator, the value may be less than, equal to, or greater than one. These fractions are called **complex fractions**.

Examples:

$$\frac{\frac{1}{4}}{4} < 1, \ \frac{\frac{1}{2}}{\frac{2}{4}} = 1, \ \frac{\frac{3}{14}}{\frac{1}{3}} > 1$$

REDUCING FRACTIONS TO LOWEST TERMS

To reduce a fraction to its lowest terms, you divide both the numerator and the denominator by the largest number that can go evenly into both.

Example:

Reduce the fraction $\frac{7}{14}$ to its lowest terms.

$$\frac{7 \div 7}{14 \div 7} = \frac{1}{2}$$

The largest number that can be used to divide both the numerator (7) and the denominator (14) is 7.

ADDING FRACTIONS

To add fractions with the same denominator, add the numerators and place the new sum over the similar denominator. Reduce and change to a mixed number if necessary.

Example:

$$\frac{1}{6} + \frac{3}{6} = \frac{1+3}{6} = \frac{4}{6}$$

Therefore, $\dfrac{4}{6} = \dfrac{\text{New numerator}}{\text{Same denominator}}$

Note: In the preceding example, the final answer can be reduced to $\dfrac{2}{3}$.

To add fractions when the denominators are not the same, find the least common denominator of each fraction. Take each new quotient and multiply it by each numerator, add the numerators, and place the new results in the proper locations.

Example:

$$\frac{1}{4} + \frac{3}{5} \text{ (the lowest common denominator is 20)}$$

You must multiply as follows:

$$\frac{1}{4} \times \frac{5}{5} = \frac{5}{20} \text{ and } \frac{3}{5} \times \frac{4}{4} = \frac{12}{20}$$

Now you can add the new fractions as follows:

$$\frac{5}{20} + \frac{12}{20} = \frac{17}{20}$$

(The result is already in lowest terms.)

SUBTRACTING FRACTIONS

To subtract fractions when the denominators are the same, subtract using only the numerators.

Example:

$$\text{Subtract} \quad \frac{7}{9} - \frac{3}{9} = \frac{7-3}{9} = \frac{4}{9}$$

Example:

$$\text{Subtract} \quad \frac{11}{6} - \frac{8}{6} = \frac{11-8}{6} = \frac{3}{6}$$

$$\text{Reduce} \quad \frac{3}{6} = \frac{1}{2}$$

To subtract fractions when the denominators are not the same, find the least common denominator.

$$\frac{5}{7} - \frac{2}{5} \quad \text{Lowest common denominator} = 35$$

Change to equal fractions.

$$\frac{5 \times 5}{7 \times 5} \quad \text{becomes} \quad \frac{25}{35}$$

$$\frac{2 \times 7}{5 \times 7} \quad \text{becomes} \quad \frac{14}{35}$$

Subtract the new numerators and place your answer over the common denominator.

$$\frac{25}{35} - \frac{14}{35} = \frac{25 - 14}{35} = \frac{11}{35}$$

MULTIPLYING FRACTIONS

To multiply fractions, multiply the numerators, multiply the denominators, and reduce the product to its lowest terms.

Example:

$$\frac{6}{8} \times \frac{4}{5} = \frac{6 \times 4}{8 \times 5} = \frac{24}{40} = \frac{3}{5}$$

To multiply a fraction by a mixed number, change the mixed number to an improper fraction before you multiply, then carry out the multiplication the same as in the preceding example.

$$3\frac{2}{4} \times \frac{2}{4}$$

Change $3\frac{2}{4}$ to $\frac{14}{4}$

Now you can multiply as before.

$$\frac{14}{4} \times \frac{2}{4} = \frac{28}{16}$$

Reduce to its lowest terms.

$$\frac{28}{16} = \frac{7}{4} = 1\frac{3}{4}$$

DIVIDING FRACTIONS

To divide a fraction by another fraction, write your problem as division, invert the divisor, multiply the fraction, and reduce.

Example:

Divide: $\dfrac{2}{3} \div \dfrac{5}{7}$

$\dfrac{2}{3}$ (dividend) $\div \dfrac{5}{7}$ (divisor)   =   quotient

$\dfrac{2}{3} \times \dfrac{7}{5}$ (inverted divisor) $\dfrac{14}{15}$

DECIMALS

- Medications are frequently ordered in decimals.

- A decimal is a fraction with a denominator that is any multiple of 10, written with a decimal point.

- A decimal's value is determined by its position to the right of the decimal point. Always add a zero (0) to the left of the decimal point for decimals that have a value which is less than 1. This helps avoid errors in reading the decimal's value (see Figure 4–2).

- When reading a decimal, it is important to remember that numbers to the right of the decimal point are fractions that have a value less than 1. Numbers to the left of the decimal point are whole numbers that have a value greater than 1. Table 4–5 shows some examples.

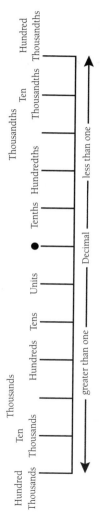

FIGURE 4–2 Understanding decimals.

Fraction	Decimal Fraction	Description

TABLE 4–5   Fractions and Their Related Decimal Fractions

Fraction	Decimal Fraction	Description
$\dfrac{4}{10}$	0.4	Because 10 has **1** zero, the decimal point of 4 is moved to the left **once**.
$\dfrac{17}{100}$	0.17	Because 100 has **2** zeros, the decimal point of 17 is moved to the left **twice**.
$\dfrac{334}{1000}$	0.334	Because 1000 has **3** zeros, the decimal point of 334 is moved to the left **three** places.

ADDING DECIMALS

To add decimals, place the decimals in a vertical column with the decimal points directly under one another. Add zeros to balance the columns. Add the decimals in the same manner used to add whole numbers, and place the decimal point in the answer under the aligned decimal points.

Example:

Add: 0.8 + 4.79 + 24

```
      0.80
      4.79
+    24.00
   -------
     29.59
```

SUBTRACTING DECIMALS

To subtract decimals, place the decimals in a vertical column with the decimal points directly under one another. Add zeros to balance the columns. Subtract the decimals in the same manner as whole numbers are subtracted, and place the decimal point in the answer under the aligned decimal points.

Example:

Subtract: 3.9 from 7.4

$$
\begin{array}{r}
7.4 \\
-\quad 3.9 \\
\hline
3.5
\end{array}
$$

MULTIPLYING DECIMALS

Multiplying by 10, 100, or 1000 is a fast and easy way to calculate dosage problems. Simply move the decimal point the same number of places to the right as there are zeros in the multiplier.

Example:

Multiply: 0.807×100

There are two zeros in the multiplier of 100. Move the decimal two places to the right, for an answer of 80.7, as shown below.

$0.807 \ = \ 0.807 \ = \ 80.7$

DIVIDING DECIMALS

To divide a decimal by a whole number, first place the decimal point in the quotient line directly above the decimal point in the dividend. Division is written using several symbols, such as $1 \div 2$ or $\frac{1}{2}$. The divisor (the number performing the division) is on the right of the first symbol.

Example:

Divide: $4.75 \div 0.5 =$

$$\frac{4.75}{0.5} = \frac{\text{Dividend}}{\text{divisor}}$$

Convert the divisor to a whole number. Move the decimal point in the dividend the same number of places to the right:

$47.5 \div 5 = 9.5$

PERCENTS, RATIOS, AND PROPORTIONS

- Percents provide a way to express the relationship of parts to a whole, similar to decimals and fractions.
- Ratios also express these relationships, and can be used to easily calculate dosages of different types of medications.
- Proportions involve the use of two equal ratios in the calculation of dosages.

PERCENTS

The term **percent** and its symbol **%** mean "hundredths." The use of percentages is common in the medical and pharmacy professions. A percent is always a division of 100.

Examples:

$$8\% \text{ means } \frac{8}{100} \text{ or } 0.08$$

$$60\% \text{ means } \frac{60}{100} \text{ or } \frac{6}{10} = 0.6$$

To change a fraction to a percent, multiply the fraction by 100, and reduce. Then, add the % symbol.

Example:

$$\frac{1}{4} = ?$$

$$\frac{1}{4} \times \frac{100}{1} = \frac{100}{4} = \frac{25}{1} = 25\%$$

RATIOS

A ratio is an expression of the relationship of a part to the whole. Ratios can be written as fractions, but are usually written in the form: A : B. The colon (:) or slash (/) is used to indicate division, and both are read as "per."

Examples:

$$1{:}4 = 1/4 = \frac{1}{4}$$

$$3{:}5 = 3/5 = \frac{3}{5}$$

PROPORTIONS

A proportion shows the relationship between two equal ratios. A proportion may be expressed as the double colon (::) or the equal symbol (=), and both are read as "as."

In colon format, the first and fourth terms are called **extremes**, and the second and third terms are called **means**.

Example:

$$2 : 4 :: 8 : 16 \quad \text{or} \quad 2 : 4 \ = \ 8 : 16$$

Convert the fractions $\dfrac{2}{4}$ and $\dfrac{8}{16}$ to a proportion. First, you must cross-multiply the numerator of the fraction on the left by the denominator of the fraction on the right:

$$2 \times 16 \ = \ 32$$

Then, multiply the denominator of the fraction on the left by the numerator of the fraction on the right:

$$4 \times 8 \ = \ 32$$

In this formula, the answer is:

$\dfrac{32}{32}$, which reduces to 1.

In the preceding example, the means and extremes are as follows:

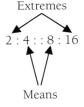

Extremes

2 : 4 :: 8 : 16

Means

To verify that two fractions are equal, cross-multiply and the products should be equal.

Example:

$$\frac{2}{5} : \frac{4}{10}$$

$$\frac{2}{5} \diagdown \!\!\!\!\!\diagup \frac{4}{10}$$

$$
\begin{aligned}
2 \times 10 &= 20 \\
5 \times 4 &= 20 \\
20 &= 20
\end{aligned}
$$

CALCULATION OF ORAL DRUGS

There are several forms of medications that are commonly administered orally. Drugs that are taken orally may be solids or liquids. Solid-form drugs are generally intended to be administered as a whole to achieve a specific effect in the body. Most tablets and capsules come in the dosage prescribed, or the order requires giving more than one pill, dividing a scored tablet in half, or mixing a dose when swallowing is difficult.

Various medications might be labeled "controlled-release," "extended-release," or "timed-release." Controlled-release drugs are intended to be released into the body in reaction to specific conditions or factors that already exist in the body. Extended-release drugs are designed to be slowly released in the body over a sustained period of time. Timed-release drugs are drugs released in small amounts over time (as by the dissolution of a coating), usually in the gastrointestinal tract.

When medications are ordered and available in the same system (for example, metric) and the same unit of size (for example, milligrams), dosage calculations are easy. When the ordered or desired dosage is different from what is available or what "you have," it is necessary to convert to the same system and the same units before calculating dosages. This can be done using either the **Ratio and Proportion Method** or the **Formula Method**.

RATIO AND PROPORTION METHOD

Example 1:

Ordered:	Codeine 15 mg p.o.
On hand:	Codeine 30 mg per tablet
Calculate:	How many tablet(s) should be given?

$$\frac{Q}{H} = \frac{X}{D} \quad \text{Or} \quad \frac{\text{Dosage unit}}{\text{Dose on hand}} = \frac{\text{Amount to be given}}{\text{Desired dose}}$$

$$\frac{1 \text{ tablet}}{30 \text{ mg}} = \frac{X}{15 \text{ mg}}$$

Cross-multiply and solve for the unknown:

$$30 \times X = 1 \text{ tablet} \times 15$$
$$X = 1 \text{ tablet} \times 15/30$$
$$X = 0.5 \text{ tablet}$$

Because 15 mg is one-half of 30 mg, $\frac{1}{2}$ tablet should be given.

FORMULA METHOD

$$\frac{D}{H} \times Q = X$$

D	=	desired amount
H	=	have available
Q	=	quantity
X	=	amount to give

Example 1:

Ordered: Keflex 80 mg p.o. q.i.d.

On hand: Keflex 250 mg per 5 mL

Calculate: How many mLs should be given?

$$\frac{D}{H} \times Q = \frac{80 \text{ mg}}{250 \text{ mg}} \times 5 \text{ mL}$$

$$\frac{80 \times 5}{250} = 1.6 \text{ mL}$$

Example 2:

Ordered: Inderal 15 mg p.o. t.i.d.

On hand: Inderal 10 mg tablets

Calculate: How many tablets should be given?

$$\frac{D}{H} \times Q = X$$

$$\frac{15 \text{ mg}}{10 \text{ mg}} \times 1 = 1.5 \text{ tablets}$$

■ CALCULATION OF PARENTERAL DOSAGES

"Parenteral" commonly refers to drug injection into body tissues (for example, SC – into fatty tissue or under skin; IM – into a muscle) and into body fluids (for example, IV – into a vein or an infusion). Injectable medications are prescribed in grams, milligrams, micrograms, grains, or units.

Small volumes of injectable drugs are given in a 3-mL syringe unless the dosage can be easily measured in a 1-mL syringe. An amount of less than 1 mL can be given in a tuberculin syringe or an insulin syringe (see Figure 4–3).

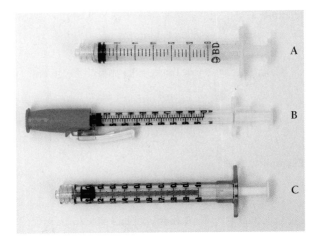

FIGURE 4–3   Types of Syringes (A) 3 cc syringe (B) Standard U-100 Insulin syringe (C) 1 mL tuberculin syringe with Luer lock.

CALCULATION OF INTRAMUSCULAR DOSAGES

For calculating intramuscular dosages, the following can be used.

Example:

Ordered: Vistaril 100 mg IM stat

On hand: Vistaril solution 50 mg/mL in a
           10-mL multiple-dose vial

By using the formula, calculate how many milli-liter(s) should be given.

$$\frac{D}{H} \times Q = \frac{100 \text{ mg}}{50 \text{ mg}} \times 1\text{mL} = 2 \text{ mL}$$

INSULIN DOSAGES

Dosage calculations for insulin are solved using units/mL. According to the onset and duration of action, insulin can be classified as: R (regular), L (lente), U (ultralente), and NPH (neutral protein Hagedorn). Due to newer insulin therapies that have increased the number of treatment options for patients, humulin ultralente and humulin lente insulins are being discontinued.

Example:

Give 40 units of insulin, using U-100 insulin. There are two different strengths of insulin, U-100 and U-500 insulin. Each patient's physician determines which strength should be used. The amount administered is calculated as follows:

$$\frac{40}{100} \times 1 \text{ mL} = 0.4 \text{ mL}$$

Portable insulin delivery devices use insulin cartridges in place of vials and syringes. Insulin pens are sometimes referred to as "dial dosage systems" because a dial is used to select the desired dose of insulin, and then a plunger is pressed to deliver the insulin into the skin.

HEPARIN DOSAGES

Heparin is an anticoagulant that prevents the formation of a new clot and the extension of an existing clot. It is obtained in unit-dose or multiple-dose vials, and in strengths ranging from 1000 to 20,000 units/mL. Heparin is prescribed in units/h or mL/h, and is administered SC or IV (for intermittent or continuous infusion) via an electronic infusion device. The patient's requirements are obtained from blood-clotting studies done initially every four hours. The normal adult heparin dosage is 20,000 to 40,000 units every 24 hours. When given IV, heparin is ordered in units per hour.

Example 1:

Ordered: heparin 6,500 units SC

On hand: heparin 10,000 units/mL

The amount to be administered is calculated as follows:

$$\text{Use } \frac{D}{H} \times Q = X$$

$$\frac{6,500}{10,000} \times 1 = 0.65 \text{ mL}$$

Example 2:

Ordered: heparin 1,000 units/h IV using an infusion pump

On hand: heparin 20,000 units in 1,500 mL of 5% DW

$$\text{Use } \frac{D}{H} \times Q = X$$

$$\frac{1,000}{20,000} \times 1500 = X$$

$$X = 75 \text{ mL/h}$$

INTRAVENOUS CALCULATIONS

Fluids can be given to a patient slowly over a period of time through a vein (intravenous) to provide fluid, nutrients, electrolytes (for example, sodium or potassium), vitamins, blood products, and specific medications to the patient. Intravenous (IV) therapy, which can be **continuous** or **intermittent**, is used for fluid replacement or fluid maintenance to treat disorders such as electrolyte imbalance, dehydration, and malnutrition.

Intravenous fluids generally contain dextrose, sodium chloride, or electrolytes:

- D/5/W (5% D/W) is a 5% dextrose solution, which means 5 grams of dextrose in 100 mL of solution.

- 0.9% NS stands for a solution in which 100 milliliters of solution contains 0.9 gram of sodium chloride.

- 5% D/O 45% NS stands for a solution containing 5 grams of dextrose in 100 milliliters of 0.45% normal saline solution.

- Ringer's lactate (RL), which is also called lactated Ringer's solution (LR), is a solution containing electrolytes.

Intravenous therapy is administered via an IV infusion set. This set consists of the following:

- IV solution
- Infusion tubing
- Drop chamber
- Control valve or clamp (roll valve)

The most commonly prescribed intravenous solutions are listed in Table 4–6.

TABLE 4–6   **Most Commonly Prescribed Intravenous Solutions**

Solution	Abbreviation
5% dextrose in water	5% D/W (D_5W)
10% dextrose in water	10% D/W ($D_{10}W$)
5% dextrose in 0.45% sodium chloride solution	$D_5 \frac{1}{2}$ NS
5% dextrose in 0.9% sodium chloride solution	5% D/0.9% NS *or* D/5/0.9% NS
Dextrose with Ringer's lactate solution	D/RL
0.45% sodium chloride solution	0.45% NS
0.9% sodium chloride solution	0.9% NS
Lactated Ringer's solution	LR, RL, *or* RLS
Lactated Ringer's and 5% dextrose solution	5% D/RL *or* D/5/RL

The drip chamber is located at the site of the entrance of the tubing into the container of IV solution. It allows the number of drops per minute that the patient is receiving (flow rate) to be counted.

A roll valve clip is connected to the tubing and can be manipulated to increase or decrease the flow rate. The **primary** IV line is either a **peripheral** line (access into the arm) or a **central** line (access into a large vein in the chest or neck). **Secondary** IV lines, also known as IV piggyback (IVPB) are used for intermittent, smaller quantity infusions (for example, a medication in 50–100 mL of fluid) and are attached to the primary line. IVPB solutions are usually given over 30–60 minutes. IVPB is always hung higher than the primary bag or bottle to allow the secondary set of medication to infuse first (see Figure 4–4).

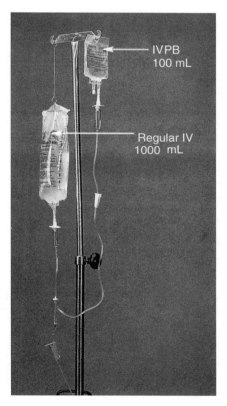

FIGURE 4–4   IV line with piggyback.

Drop Factor

Manufacturers specify the number of drops that equal 1 milliliter for their particular tubing. This equivalent is called the tubing's **drop factor** or **calibration**.

Calculation of Intravenous Flow Rates

A flow rate is the speed at which IV fluids are infused into a patient. The ability of the pharmacy technician to correctly and efficiently calculate flow rates of IV fluids is critical to the well-being of the patient.

Flow rates are commonly prescribed as 125 mL/hr or 500 mL/2 hr, meaning that fluids should be infused into the patient at a rate of 125 mL over a period of 1 hour, or at a rate of 500 mL over a period of 2 hours. Flow rates can be controlled either by the use of an electronic pump, or by manually adjusting the intravenous equipment to achieve the physician's order for flow rate.

If an electronic pump is used, the following formula can be utilized:

$$\frac{\text{Total amount ordered (mL)}}{\text{Total number of hours (hr)}} = \text{mL/hr}$$

Example:

500 mL bag of IV fluids to be infused over 2 hours:

By using the preceding formula, the flow rate can be calculated:

$$\frac{500 \text{ mL}}{2 \text{ hr}} = 250 \text{ mL/hr}$$

Manually Calculating Drop Rates

To calculate the drop rate, the technician must determine how many drops (abbreviated as *gtt*) per minute should be infused over a prescribed time period. The number of drops per minute depends on the type of IV tubing used. Two types of tubing are available: macrodrip and microdrip (see Table 4–7).

The drop factor is generally found on the outside packaging of the tubing and indicates the number of drops per milliliter a particular IV tubing set will deliver (see Figure 4–5).

This formula is used to calculate flow rates in drops per minute:

$$\frac{V}{T} \times C = R$$

V = total volume to be infused in mL
T = total time in minutes
C = drop factor in gtt/mL
R = rate of flow in gtt/min

TABLE 4–7	Common Drop Factors
Macrodrip	Microdrip
10 gtt/mL	60 gtt/mL
15 gtt/mL	90 gtt/mL
20 gtt/mL	120 gtt/mL

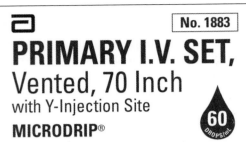

FIGURE 4–5 The drop factor can be found on the packaging of the IV tubing. *(Courtesy of Abbott Laboratories, Inc.)*

Example:

A patient is to receive 400 mL of IV fluids over 2 hours. Macrodrip tubing has been selected (a drop factor of 20 gtt/min). The technician wants to calculate how many drops per minute are needed.

Step 1:   Convert 2 hours into minutes
(remember: 1 hour = 60 minutes)

$$2 \times 60 = 120 \text{ minutes}$$

Step 2:   Use the formula:

$$\frac{V}{T} \times C = R$$

$$\frac{400}{120} \times 20 = 66.6 \text{ or } 67 \text{ gtt/min}$$

■ PEDIATRIC DOSAGE CALCULATIONS

Three formulas are used to calculate dosages for infants and children. They are as follows:

- Young's rule
- Clark's rule
- Fried's rule

These rules give only approximate dosages. Even when pediatric drug dosages are calculated on the basis of body surface area, weight, and age of the child, they are based on a proportion of the usual adult dose (approximate).

YOUNG'S RULE

Infants and children are more sensitive to medications than are adults. Their age, weight, height, and the immature function of some of their organs (such as the liver and kidneys) may be major factors. Dosage must be calculated accurately according to the age and weight of infants and children. Young's rule is used for children older than 1 year of age, but not older than 12 years of age.

$$\text{Pediatric dose} = \frac{\text{Child's age in years}}{\text{Child's age in years} + 12} \times \text{Adult dose}$$

Example:

Calculate the dose of phenobarbital for a 2-year-old child (adult dose = 600 mg):

$$\frac{2 \text{ (years)}}{2 \text{ (years)} + 12} \times 600 \quad = \quad \frac{2 \times 600}{14}$$

$$\frac{1200}{14} \quad = \quad 86 \text{ mg}$$

Remember...

Young's rule is not valid for children older than 12 years of age.

CLARK'S RULE

Clark's rule is based on the weight of the child. This system is much more accurate than other pediatric methods, because the size and body weight of children of any age can vary greatly. Clark's rule uses 150 pounds (70 kg) as the average adult weight and assumes that the child's dose is proportionately less.

$$\text{Pediatric dose} \quad = \quad \frac{\text{Child's weight in pounds}}{150 \text{ pounds}} \times \text{Adult dose}$$

Example:

Calculate the dose of furosemide (Lasix) for a 45-pound child.

(adult dose = 80 mg in 1 dose)

$$\frac{45}{150} \times 80 \quad = \quad 24 \text{ mg}$$

FRIED'S RULE

Fried's rule is a method of estimating the dose of medication for infants younger than 1 year of age.

$$\frac{\text{Age in months}}{150} \times \text{average adult dose} = \text{child's dose}$$

Example:

Calculate the dose of digoxin for an 11-month-old infant.

(adult dose = 1 mg in divided doses over 24-hr)

$$\frac{11}{150} \times 1 \text{ mg} = 0.07\text{mg}$$

CALCULATE DOSAGE BASED ON BODY SURFACE AREA (BSA)

Body surface area is the most accurate way to determine the amount of a drug to be administered to a child. To calculate a pediatric dosage based on body surface area, divide the child's body surface area in square meters (m^2) (by using the nomogram in Figure 4–6) by 1.73 m^2 (the surface area of an average adult), and then multiply by the adult dose. For practical use, the adult body surface area is sometimes rounded to 1.7 m^2.

Pediatric dose =

$$\frac{\text{Body surface area (BSA) of the child in } m^2}{1.7 \text{ } m^2 \text{ (average adult BSA)}} \times \text{Adult dose}$$

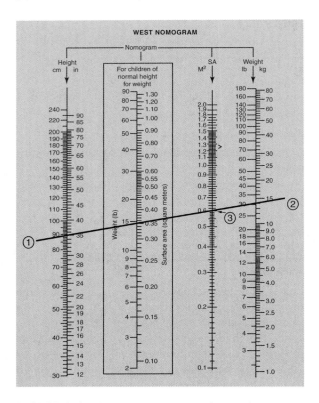

FIGURE 4–6 The West nomogram. *(From Behrman, RE, Kliegman, RM, Jenson, HB, (Eds): Nelson Textbook of Pediatrics, 16th ed. Philadelphia: WB Saunders, 2000. Reprinted with permission.)*

Example:

The child's BSA is 0.84 m². The recommended dosage is 0.4 mg/m². Determine the child's dose.

$$\text{Pediatric dose} = \frac{0.84 \text{ m}^2}{1.7 \text{ m}^2} \times 0.4 \text{ mg/m}^2$$

$$\frac{0.84 \times 0.4}{1.7} = \frac{0.336}{1.7}$$

$$\text{Pediatric dose} = 0.20 \text{ mg}$$

■ ALLIGATION ALTERNATE

Alligation alternate is an arithmetic method used to determine what quantities of two or more preparations of differing strengths to mix to achieve a final product of the desired quantity and strength. The strengths of mixtures used in alligation-alternate calculations are usually expressed in terms of percentage strengths.

The quantities produced by these calculations are usually expressed in parts, which can be used to calculate actual amounts in grams or milliliters. The strengths of a mixture of preparations lie somewhere between the strengths of the weaker and stronger components, but is always nearer to the strength of the component present in greater quantity.

The following figure is used to determine the relative proportion of components to mix together to achieve a product of the desired percentage strength.

Example:

In what proportion should a 95% preparation and a 50% preparation be mixed to make a 70% solution?

Note the *difference* between the strength of the stronger component (95%) and the desired strength used (that is, 25 parts). The difference between the desired strength (70%) and the strength of the weaker component (50%) indicates the number of parts of the stronger to be used (that is, 20 parts).

Thus, the proportion or ratio of the 95% and 50% preparations to use in making a 70% solution is 20 : 25, a *total* of 45 parts. The ratio may be reduced to 4 : 5, with a total of 9 parts.

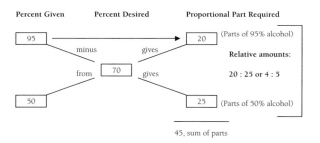

Percent Given   **Percent Desired**   **Proportional Part Required**

| 95 | | 20 | (Parts of 95% alcohol) |

minus   gives

Relative amounts:

from   70   gives   **20 : 25 or 4 : 5**

| 50 | | 25 | (Parts of 50% alcohol) |

45, sum of parts

5

Prescriptions

A **prescription** is an order for medication issued by a
physician, dentist, or other properly licensed medical
practitioner. Various states also license other prescribers
who have limited scope of practice. In some states, nurse
practitioners, optometrists, psychologists, and even pharmacists can issue prescriptions under protocol or with certain
restrictions. Prescriptions designate a specific medication
and dosage to be administered to a particular patient at a
specific time. ■

THE PRESCRIPTION ORDER FORM

Prescriptions are usually written on printed forms that
contain blank spaces for the required information.
They may be either in the form of prescription blanks
or hospital medication orders.

PRESCRIPTION BLANKS

Prescription blanks are supplied in the form of a pad.
Most prescription blanks are imprinted with the name,

address, telephone number, and other pertinent information of the physician or his or her practice site (clinic or hospital) (see Figure 5–1).

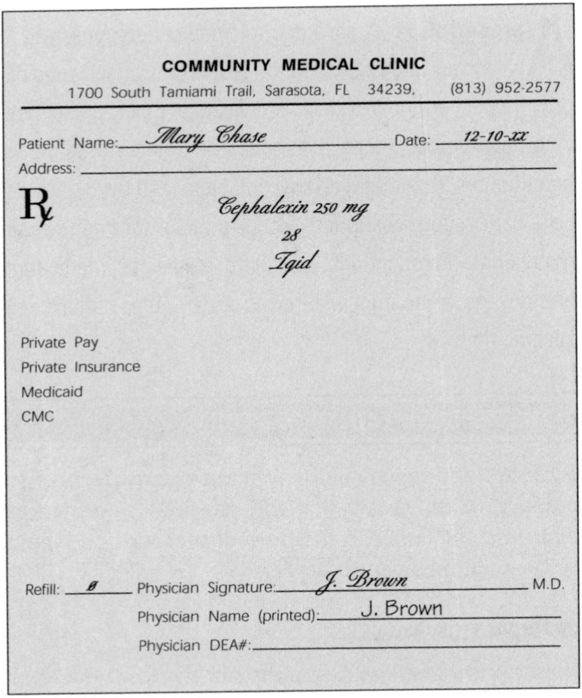

COMMUNITY MEDICAL CLINIC
1700 South Tamiami Trail, Sarasota, FL 34239, (813) 952-2577

Patient Name: _Mary Chase_ Date: _12-10-xx_
Address: _____

℞ *Cephalexin 250 mg*
28
Tqid

Private Pay
Private Insurance
Medicaid
CMC

Refill: _0_ Physician Signature: _J. Brown_ M.D.
Physician Name (printed): _J. Brown_
Physician DEA#: _____

FIGURE 5–1 **Prescription.**

HOSPITAL MEDICATION ORDERS

A medication order for an inpatient in a hospital or other institution is written by the physician on a form called a **Physician's Order Sheet**. The type of form used varies between institutions and even within an institution, depending on the unit rendering the care (see Figure 5–2). For additional information in medication orders see Chapter 8.

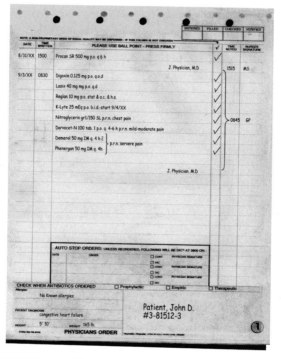

FIGURE 5–2   Physician's order.

■ PARTS OF THE PRESCRIPTION

Every prescription has four basic parts: the super-scription, inscription, subscription, and signature.

- **Superscription**—the date, the patient's full name and address, date of birth, and the symbol ℞, which means "take thou" in Latin
- **Inscription**—the name of the drug, amount, and concentration
- **Subscription**—the directions to the pharmacist
- **Signature**, or **transcription**—patient instructions

  A prescription also includes these items:
- Physician's name, office address and telephone number, and D.E.A. registration number
- Physician's signature
- Number of times the prescription can be refilled
- Indication of whether the pharmacist may substitute a generic version of a trade name drug at the patient's request (See Figure 5–1.)

■ PROCESSING THE PRESCRIPTION ORDER

Proper procedures are given in the following sections for the important tasks that a pharmacist or technician must accomplish in the processing of a prescription order. These include receiving, reading and checking, numbering and dating, labeling, preparing, packaging, rechecking, delivering, counseling, recording and filing, and pricing.

RECEIVING THE PRESCRIPTION

The pharmacy technician must do the following:

- Gather essential disease and drug information.
- Obtain the correct name, address, and other pertinent patient information.
- Determine the patient's medication insurance coverage.
- Ask the patient if he or she wishes to wait, wants a call back, or wants the medication delivered.

Methods of Receiving a Prescription

A prescription may arrive via the following:

- Written Prescription: The technician is able to receive a written prescription from the customer.
- Telephone: Only a licensed pharmacist can receive the prescription by phone.
- Fax: The technician is able to receive a prescription via fax. Schedule II drugs must have a written prescription followed up at the pharmacy within 72 hours.
- Voice mail.
- E-mail (utilizing *e-scribe* or *pre-scribe* software).

It is important to know the rules and regulations in your state of practice regarding receipt of prescriptions. As new technologies develop, the federal and state requirements are revised. It is important to stay abreast of the latest rules and regulations.

READING AND CHECKING THE PRESCRIPTION

The pharmacy technician should do the following:

- Read the prescription completely and carefully.
- Determine the compatibility of the newly prescribed medication with other drugs being taken by the patient.
- Consider if any drug-food or drug-disease interactions may exist.

NUMBERING AND DATING

The pharmacy technician is required legally to do the following:

- Number the prescription order.
- Place the same number on the label.
- Date the prescription with the date it is filled.

LABELING

The prescription label may be typewritten or prepared by computer using the information entered by the pharmacist or pharmacy technician. Figure 5–3 shows a computer-prepared prescription and label. Newer laser printers produce a label with a typeface and boldness that is much easier for most patients to read.

The following is legally required to appear on the prescription label:

- Name and address of the pharmacy; the telephone number is also commonly included.

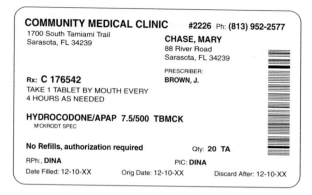

FIGURE 5–3   Computer-prepared prescription and label.

- Prescription number.
- Prescriber's name.
- Patient's name.
- Directions for use.
- The date of dispensing.
- The name and strength of the medication are not required but frequently included. Auxiliary labels are available in various colors to give them special prominence.

Examples of some auxiliary labels are shown in Figure 5–4.

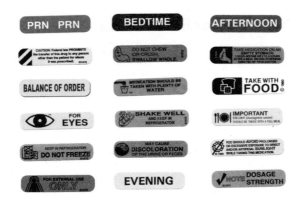

FIGURE 5–4   Auxiliary labels.

PREPARING THE PRESCRIPTION

The pharmacist or the technician must decide the exact procedure to be followed in dispensing or compounding the ingredients.

PACKAGING

When dispensing a prescription, pharmacy technicians should:

- Select an appropriate container from various shapes, sizes, colors, and composition.

- By law, prescription containers must be moisture proof. Selection is based primarily on the type and quantity of medication to be dispensed, and the method of its use.

Types of containers generally used in the pharmacy include:

- **Prescription bottles:** used for dispensing liquids of low viscosity
- **Round vials:** used primarily for solid dosage forms such as capsules and tablets
- **Dropper bottles:** used for dispensing ophthalmic, nasal, otic, or oral liquids to be administered by drops
- **Ointment jars:** used to dispense semisolid dosage forms such as creams and ointments

Figure 5–5 shows some examples of the different types of containers available.

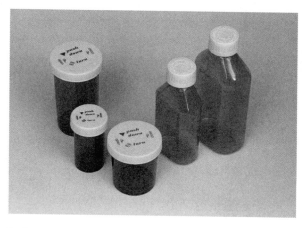

FIGURE 5–5   Various medication containers for dispensing.

Child-Resistant Containers

The high number of accidental poisonings of children after ingestion of medications and other household chemicals led to the passage of the *Poison Prevention Packaging Act*. The act's initial regulation called for use of *childproof* closures for aspirin products and certain household chemicals. Effective closures for these containers were developed, and the regulations were extended to include the use of such safety closures in the packaging of both legend and over-the-counter (OTC) medications.

RECHECKING

Before giving a prescription to the patient, every prescription should be rechecked. This is done by:

- The pharmacist verifying the ingredients and amounts used
- Reviewing all details of the label against the prescription order to verify directions, patient's name, prescription number, date, and prescriber's name

DELIVERING

The pharmacist should personally present the prescription medication to the patient or his or her family member unless it is to be delivered to the patient's home or workplace by the pharmacy technician.

PATIENT COUNSELING

The pharmacist should personally reinforce the information the physician has already provided the patient.

There is an increased awareness that labeling instructions frequently are inadequate to ensure patient understanding of his or her medication. The prescriber and the pharmacist share the responsibility that the patient receives specific instructions, precautions, and warnings for safe and effective use of prescribed drugs.

RECORDING AND FILING

A record of the prescriptions dispensed is maintained in the pharmacy through the use of computer and hard-copy prescription files. Newer centralized computer systems used by many chain drugstores allow pharmacists from any location to access a patient's records in the system, and refill a prescription previously dispensed at another store.

Various prescription file types are available to maintain original prescription orders. Metal or cardboard units, which conveniently store approximately 1000 prescriptions, are common. When these files are used, holes are punched in the prescription orders; the files are then slipped onto tiny, firmly attached metal rods and placed in a designated compartment in numerical order for safe storage and rapid retrieval. It is important that the technician document and record that the prescription arrived to the pharmacy by telephone, fax, voice mail, as a written prescription, or in an e-mail.

PRICING THE PRESCRIPTION

For a prescription practice to be successful, the pharmacist must make a fair and equitable profit. Each pharmacy should have a method for pricing prescriptions that is applied consistently by each pharmacist practicing in the pharmacy. The pricing method should be established to ensure the profitable operation of the prescription department, as well as providing a reasonable margin of profit on investment.

■ PRESCRIPTION REFILLING

Instructions for refilling a prescription are provided by the prescriber on the original prescription, or by verbal communication. Although prescriptions for non-controlled substances have no limitation according to federal law as to the number of refills permitted, or the date of expiration, state laws may impose such limits. Refilling prescriptions for controlled substances is limited, and both the original and transferred prescription drug order shall be maintained for a period of five years from the date of the last refill.

6

Dosage Forms and Administration of Medications

The route of administration, in part, regulates drug action. Serious drug errors and death can result when a drug is delivered by the wrong route. Each member of the health-care team involved in medication administration must be constantly vigilant to prevent errors and deliver quality patient care. The health-care team must be familiar with many different forms of medications, as well as with their routes of administration, doses, and strengths. A medication should never be given until its purpose, possible side effects, precautions, and recommended dosages are known. ■

■ THE SEVEN RIGHTS OF MEDICATION ADMINISTRATION

- Right patient
- Right drug
- Right dose
- Right time
- Right route

- Right technique
- Right documentation

DRUG FORMS

Drug dosage forms are classified according to their physical state and chemical composition. During manufacturing, the drug itself is mixed with other substances to create the form needed. The nontherapeutic substance is called the **vehicle**. This vehicle is the substance added to a drug to give the drug bulk or suitable consistency, and may be a solid, semisolid, liquid, or gas.

SOLID DRUGS

Solid drugs include tablets, pills, plasters, capsules, caplets, gelcaps, powders, granules, troches, or lozenges. Solid drugs are generally administered via the oral route.

SEMISOLID DRUGS

Semisolid drugs include suppositories, ointments, and gels. Semisolid drugs are often used as topical applications. These drugs are soft and pliable.

LIQUID DRUGS

Liquid preparations include drugs that have been dissolved or suspended. Examples of liquid drugs are syrups, spirits, elixirs, tinctures, fluidextracts, liniments, emulsions, solutions, mixtures, suspensions, aromatic waters, sprays, and aerosols. Liquid drugs may be administered systemically by mouth or injected, by using different techniques, into the skin, muscles, or veins.

GASES

Gases are a basic form of matter that has no discernable shape or volume. Pharmaceutical gases include:

- Anesthetic gases (nitrous oxide)
- Compressed gases (oxygen for therapy, or carbon dioxide)

  Gases are generally administered through inhalation.

■ PRINCIPLES OF DRUG ADMINISTRATION

The pharmacy technician must know the correct administrative route for any drug that is required. The chosen route of drug administration determines the rate and intensity of the drug's effect.

ORAL ADMINISTRATION

Oral administration is by the mouth, abbreviated as PO (per os). The oral route is the easiest and most common route of medication administration. It is also the safest and the most acceptable to patients. The pharmacy technician should be aware of the following when administering drugs by the oral route:

- Water is contraindicated when giving medications intended for local effects, such as cough syrup and lozenges, or when giving buccal or sublingual medications, which are absorbed locally for a systemic effect and must not be swallowed.
- If the patient has trouble swallowing, a large swallow of water before taking the pill or capsule may moisten the oral mucosa and make swallowing easier. Drinking through a straw or bottle with a

narrow neck may make solid forms of medication easier to swallow.

- If the dosage requires that a scored tablet be broken, use a gauze square for breaking. Never break the tablet using bare hands.
- Never crush enteric tablets because the strongly acidic contents of the stomach can destroy some medications. These **enteric-coated** tablets are designed to dissolve in the small intestine.
- Never open or crush extended, controlled release, or time-release capsules. This is because sustained-release tablets or capsules are designed to dissolve very slowly.
- Keep all medications out of the reach of children.

PARENTERAL ADMINISTRATION

Parenteral administration refers to dispensing drugs by routes other than oral or topical, and the delivery of medications via a needle into the:

- Skin layers
- Subcutaneous tissue
- Muscles
- Veins

Drugs are administered parenterally for the following reasons:

1. The medication effect is required quickly.
2. The patient cannot take an oral medication.

3. Gastric acid or enzymes might destroy the medication.

4. The drug might be prematurely removed from the body on a "first pass" through the liver.

5. The medication preparation is not available in an enteral form.

6. The medication must be given at a controlled rate to achieve a continuous blood level.

There are four main categories for parenteral administration, according to the site of injection. Drugs may be injected into muscles (intramuscular), skin (intradermal or subcutaneous), veins (intravenous), and the spinal column (intrathecal). Table 6–1 lists needles and syringes for different types of injections.

Basic Equipment for Parenteral Administration

Administration of drugs by injection requires basic equipment:

- Needles
  - Disposable or nondisposable
  - Gauges commonly range in size from 16 to 30
  - Lengths commonly vary from $\frac{3}{8}$ to 2 inches
- Syringes
  - Disposable or nondisposable
  - Sizes include 1, 3, 5, 10, 20, and 50 mL
  - Types of syringes include hypodermic, insulin, tuberculin, needleless, prefilled, and injector pen
  - Gauge size varies

Medication Containers

Medications prescribed for injection are available in different containers, such as ampules, vials, and sterile cartridges with premeasured medications.

Intradermal Injections

- An intradermal medication is injected into the dermal layer of the skin, the superficial layer of skin just below the epidermis.

- Injections are made into the inner aspect of the forearm, which is the common site. Other sites that may be used are the upper chest and back.

- The angle of insertion is 15 degrees.

- Skin tests for allergies and tuberculin tests are the most common uses for intradermal injections (see Figure 6–1).

Subcutaneous Injections

- Subcutaneous injections involve placing no more than 2 mL of medication fluid into the layer of fatty tissue called adipose tissue.

- Because there is normally less blood supplied to adipose tissue than to muscle, any medication injected into that tissue will be slowly, but completely, absorbed. This produces a relatively slow onset of medication action, but a long drug action.

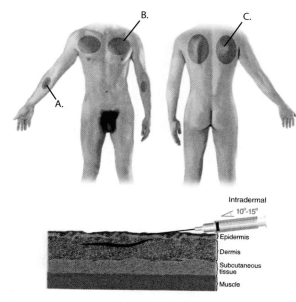

FIGURE 6–1 **Intradermal injection sites and needle angle.**

- Medications injected into the subcutaneous tissue are usually very strong, but concentrated into small doses. For example, the drugs most frequently given subcutaneously are insulin and heparin.

- The most common sites for subcutaneous injections are the deltoid area, anterior thigh, abdomen, and upper back. The angle of insertion is 45 degrees for local anesthetics, allergy treatments, and epinephrine (see Figure 6–2).

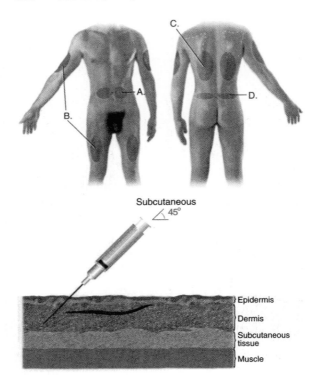

FIGURE 6–2   Subcutaneous injections sites and needle angle.

Intramuscular Injections

- The intramuscular route is a common route for parenteral injections.

- Many antibiotics, vaccines, preoperative sedatives, and narcotics are administered intramuscularly.

- With intramuscular injections, the medication is deposited deep into the muscle mass. Because the muscles contain large blood vessels and nerves, it is important to correctly place the needle to avoid damage.

- The preferred sites are the gluteus, deltoid, and vastus lateralis muscles of the adult. The vastus lateralis is the safest site of administration for infants.

- The angle of insertion is 90 degrees.

- The volume of medication may vary from 0.5 to 5 mL. In adults, up to 2 to 3 mL is recommended. Only 1 mL of medication can be injected into the deltoid muscle, whereas up to 5 mL can be injected into the gluteal site. Infants and children should be given no more than 2 mL in the vastus lateralis or ventrogluteal sites (see Figure 6–3).

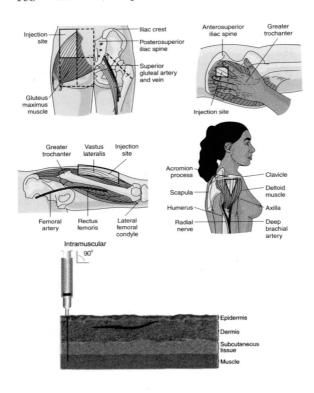

FIGURE 6–3   Intramuscular injection sites and needle angle.

Intravenous Injections

- The **intravenous route** is used when it is necessary for medication to enter the blood circulation directly.

- Sometimes, large doses of medication must be administered, either every few hours or over a long period of time. Because IV medication has not been exposed to other enzymes or tissues before reaching the blood circulation, the rate of absorption and the onset of action are faster. In emergencies, medication may be injected directly into a vein, but usually the IV medication is given on a scheduled basis, or infused slowly through IV tubing or an infusion line that is already in the vein. In most instances, a nurse performs the initial **venipuncture**, or insertion of a needle into a vein. The peripheral veins for intravenous therapy are shown in Figure 6–4.

TABLE 6–1   Selection of Needles and Syringes

Route	Gauge	Length (in.)	Volume to Be Injected (mL)
Intradermal	25–27 G	$\frac{3}{8} - \frac{1}{2}$	0.01–0.1 mL
Subcutaneous	25–27 G	$\frac{1}{2} - 1$	0.5–2 mL
Intramuscular	20–22 G	1–2	0.5–2 mL
Intravenous	15–22 G	$\frac{1}{2} - 2$	Unlimited

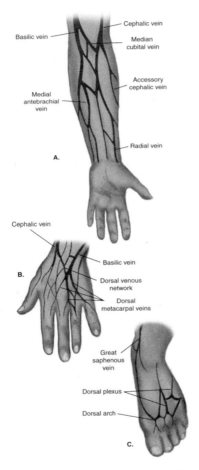

FIGURE 6–4 **Peripheral veins used for intravenous injections (A) Arm and forearm; (B) Dorsum of the hand; (C) Dorsal plexus of the foot.**

Spinal Anesthesia

Spinal anesthesia is a method of administering a local anesthetic into the spinal column. This deadens sensations from the point of administration down to the feet.

PERCUTANEOUS ADMINISTRATION

- Percutaneous administration is the application of medication for absorption through the mucous membranes or skin. Many drugs are now administered through transdermal systems to provide broad systemic effects.

- Medication administered percutaneously acts locally to cleanse, soften, disinfect, or lubricate the skin. The amount of medication absorbed through the skin or mucous membranes depends on the following factors:

  - The concentration or strength of the drug
  - The size of the area covered by medication
  - The length of time the medication stays in contact with the skin
  - Hydration status
  - Condition of the skin

- Percutaneous routes include the following:

  - Applying topical creams, powders, ointments, or lotions
  - Putting solutions onto the mucous membranes of the ear, eye, nose, mouth, rectum, or vagina
  - Inhaling aerosolized liquids or gases to carry medication to nasal passages, sinuses, and lungs

Topical Route

Topical medications are applied directly to the area of skin requiring treatment. The most common forms of topical medications include creams, lotions, and ointments, although there are many others.

Transdermal Patches

Certain medications can be absorbed slowly through the skin to create a constant, time-released systemic effect. For example, transdermal patches are dosage forms that release minute amounts of drug at a consistent rate. Examples of drugs administered transdermally include nitroglycerin, estrogen, nicotine, testosterone, and scopolamine.

Sublingual Administration

Sublingual administration is when the patient places the tablet under the tongue until completely dissolved. Medication is rapidly absorbed through the blood capillaries and enters the systemic circulation. This site is used for nitroglycerin tablets to relieve chest pain.

Buccal Administration

Buccal administration is when the patient holds the medication between the cheek and gum until it is dissolved. It is rapidly absorbed into the blood circulation. The buccal route is preferred over the sublingual route for sustained-release delivery because of its greater mucosal surface area.

Inhalation Administration

Medication may be sent into the lungs by using aerosol nebulizers, or metered-dose inhalers. Medications that are administered through inhalers include bronchodilators, mucolytic agents, and steroids. Metered-dose inhalers deliver medication in an inert propellant gas, and require good hand-breath coordination.

Ophthalmic Administration

Sterile drops or ointments in very low dosages may be administered into the eyes. The medications are placed between the eyeball and the lower eyelid (see Figure 6–5).

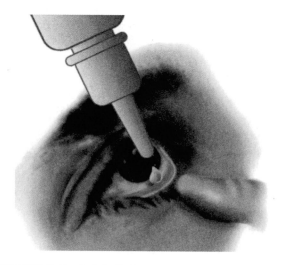

FIGURE 6–5 Ophthalmic route.

Medications in ophthalmic preparations include antibiotics, antivirals, decongestants, artificial tears, and topical anesthetics.

Otic Administration

The otic route is used to treat local conditions of the ear, including infections and soft blockages of the auditory canal. Otic medications include eardrops and irrigations, which are usually ordered for cleaning purposes. Administration to infants and young children must be performed carefully to avoid injury to sensitive structures of the ear.

Nasal Administration

The nasal route is used both for local and for systemic drug administration. Nasal spray formulations of corticosteroids have revolutionized the treatment of allergic rhinitis due to their high safety margin when administered by this route. However, patients often misuse nasal decongestant sprays and nasal drops. Because rebound congestion can occur with overuse, sprays and drops should not be used for more than five days. Nasal medications are commonly used for blocked nasal passages (decongestants) and nosebleeds. Nasal administration differs from the inhalation route because nasally administered medications have localized effects, and are not delivered deeply into the lungs.

Vaginal Administration

The vaginal route is used to deliver medications to treat local infections and to relieve vaginal pain and itching. Medications are deposited into the vagina. Local contraceptives are available as creams and foams. Vaginal instillation is most effective if the patient is lying down. Creams are instilled with applicators.

Rectal Administration

The rectal route may be used for either local or systemic drug administration. It is a safe and effective means of delivering drugs to patients who are nauseated, vomiting, or comatose. Rectal drugs are normally in suppository form, although a few laxative and diagnostic agents are given via enema.

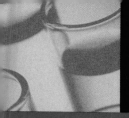

Section II

Community and Institutional Pharmacy

7

Community or Retail Pharmacy

The term **community pharmacy** is also known as **retail pharmacy**. This type of pharmacy setting provides pharmaceuticals and pharmaceutical care services to patients and the general public. There are two main categories: chain pharmacies and independent pharmacies. Independent pharmacies may also be part of a franchise, similar to chain pharmacies.

The most important functions of pharmacists in the community pharmacy include:

1. Distribution of prescribed drug products
2. Computerized connection between pharmacies across the nation involving all drugs that are legally available
3. Compounding prescriptions
4. Consulting with and educating patients ▪

DUTIES OF THE PHARMACY TECHNICIAN IN THE COMMUNITY PHARMACY

The pharmacy technician now has more responsibilities than ever before. These duties include:

- Processing the prescription
- Record keeping
- Pricing
- Answering telephone calls
- Computer applications in the control of drug use
- Accountability
- Maintaining privacy
- Communication skills
- Teamwork
- Purchasing
- Inventory control
- Billing
- Repackaging products
- Preventing drug errors
- Safe methods of working

PRESCRIPTION PROCESSING

The pharmacy technician's duties related to processing each prescription are outlined in Chapter 5.

RECORD KEEPING

The patient's record can be used in the following ways:

- Continuity of care among health-care providers
- Filing insurance claims
- Resolving legal matters such as lawsuits
- Patient information, which contains:
  - Demographics
  - Billing information
  - Social Security numbers
  - Addresses
  - Phone numbers
  - Marital status
  - Insurance carriers
  - Health history (allergies, etc.)
  - Medication log (lists), including OTC drugs and herbal preparations

PRICING

The pharmacy technician must assist in the financial aspects of the pharmacy business to maintain and make a fair profit. The charge applied to a prescription should cover the costs of the ingredients, which include:

- Containers and labels
- Time of the pharmacist or technician and auxiliary personnel involved

- Cost of inventory maintenance
- Operation costs of the pharmacy

ANSWERING PHONE CALLS

The pharmacy technician is required to conduct much of the pharmacy's daily business over the telephone. When speaking with a caller, remember the following key points:

- Always identify yourself and the pharmacy.
- Be as courteous over the telephone as you would be with someone face to face.
- Listen attentively and do not interrupt callers until they finish.
- Think about how the caller feels.
- Ask questions if you do not understand something.
- Listen for overtones (learn from a person's tone of voice and rate of speech).
- Take notes to help you remember the important points (especially dates and times).
- Give clear explanations.
- Try to avoid placing callers on hold.

COMPUTER APPLICATIONS IN THE CONTROL OF DRUG USE

Computers assist staff members in the pharmacy in the following ways:

- Performing repetitive tasks
- Reducing medication errors
- Speeding up production
- Recalling information on command

- Saving time
- Reducing paperwork and storage space
- Allowing for more creative and productive use of workers' time
- Accessing online software programs
- Allowing free downloads of software
- Computerized inventory systems
- Ordering systems (automated ordering)
- Automated dispensing systems, such as:
  - Backer Cells
  - Pyxis Supply Station
  - Homerus

ACCOUNTABILITY

Pharmacy technicians must realize the limitations and boundaries of what they can or cannot do legally. They must be accountable for their performance and also for their mistakes. An error, even a small one, can be dangerous and even life threatening for a client or a customer. Errors can also cause legal problems for the pharmacy itself. Pharmacy technicians must always strive to ensure accuracy and accountability in their job tasks. It is important to remember to double-check everything that is done to avoid errors.

MAINTAINING PRIVACY

The importance of confidentiality in the medical environment cannot be stressed enough. Patients are entitled to privacy where their health is concerned.

COMMUNICATION SKILLS

Communication is a very important factor for pharmacy technicians. They must be able to communicate with patients, customers, pharmacy staff, and other health-care professionals to serve their combined needs. A constructive pharmacist-patient relationship is essential to sound health-care practice and the optimal well-being of the patient. These relationships begin and develop with effective communication, both verbal and nonverbal. Examples of nonverbal communication include:

- Eye contact
- Facial expressions
- Hand gestures
- Grooming and dress
- Spacial awareness
- Tone of voice
- Posture
- Physical contact

TEAMWORK

Staff members must work together for the good of the patients they serve. The following are important factors of good teamwork:

- All team members must enjoy working in the pharmacy.
- Everyone likes and gets along with every other employee.

- Personal feelings must be set aside at work.
- All staff members must cooperate with others to get the job done efficiently.

PURCHASING

The pharmacy technician may order products for use or sale. The pharmacy technician may deal directly with purchasing agents and pharmaceutical or medical supply companies on matters such as pricing. It is important to follow the guidelines and policy of the pharmacy at all times. Purchase-order forms that include product name, amount, and price must be filled out and completed correctly. Remember that selection of drugs must always remain the responsibility of the pharmacist. Schedule II drugs can only be ordered by the PIC or pharmacist possessing power of attorney.

INVENTORY CONTROL

When supplies or pharmaceutical products are received, the technician must carefully check the product against the purchase order, packing slip, or invoice. All damaged products must be reported without delay and returned to the manufacturer. Another responsibility of the technician is to check all products for expiration dates.

BILLING RECORDS

Pharmacy technicians should be familiar with:

- Billing procedures and different types of insurance
- Third-party policies (HMOs and insurance)

- Information on completing insurance forms
- Authorization of third-party transactions
- Processing credit cards electronically

REPACKAGING PRODUCTS

The repackaging of pharmaceutical products usually involves unit dose medications. Repackaged medications must be properly labeled. Expiration dates must be verified. Repackaging may only be conducted by licensed pharmacists or pharmacy personnel who are allowed to conduct such activities under the laws of their state.

PREVENTING DRUG ERRORS

Medication errors may be made in prescribing, dispensing, or administering. The following factors may result in drug errors:

- Wrong drug
- Wrong dose
- Wrong time
- Wrong technique
- Wrong route
- Wrong information on the patient's chart

   Other factors that may cause errors include:

- Difficulty in reading handwritten orders
- Confusion about different drugs with similar names
- Different brand names for the same generic name
- Lack of information about a patient's drug allergies

SAFE METHODS OF WORKING

The importance of safety in the pharmacy cannot be overemphasized. Using safe practices in the pharmacy requires a personal commitment and concern for others. Pharmacy hazards include:

- Physical hazards, such as:
  - Electrical hazards
  - Fire hazards
  - Mechanical hazards
- Chemical hazards, such as:
  - Caustic chemicals
  - Poisonous chemicals
  - Carcinogenic chemicals
  - Teratogenic chemicals

ORGANIZATION OF THE RETAIL PHARMACY

All areas of the pharmacy are designed to achieve a particular goal in providing services. The floor plan of the majority of retail pharmacies includes the following:

1. Prescription counter
2. Transaction windows (drive-through windows)
3. Storage of completed prescriptions
4. Computer systems
5. Equipment for filling, labeling, and packaging; including robotic machinery
6. Refrigerator
7. Customer pick-up

8. Cash register
9. A locked storage cabinet for controlled substances
10. Consultation area
11. Sink
12. Storage area

CUSTOMER SERVICES AREA

Technicians in the community pharmacy interact with patients as customers. The customer service area is one of the most important aspects of the community pharmacy. The pharmacy technician must be skilled in communicating with patients and other customers.

CUSTOMER PICKUP

Many customers pick up their prescriptions in the customer service area. Many community pharmacies also have drive-through windows to permit customers or patients to drop off, purchase, and pick up their medications.

CASH REGISTER

The technician may be required to deal with the cash register and accept payments from patients for prescriptions or other items at the pharmacy. Cash register machines are connected to the pharmacy's computer system and can provide prices automatically by using barcode scanners.

STORAGE CABINETS FOR CONTROLLED SUBSTANCES

It is wise to keep controlled substances in a locked storage cabinet that is under the pharmacist's supervision.

The pharmacy technician must take direction from the pharmacist about which controlled substances he or she may handle in preparation for distribution to customers.

REFRIGERATOR

All pharmacies must have a refrigerator to store drugs that must be kept at a temperature between 36° to 46°F (or 2 to 8°C). The refrigerator must be used exclusively for medications. No food or beverages are allowed to be stored in any refrigerator in which medications are stored. Pharmacy technicians should check the refrigerator temperature daily and document the temperature. It is important to note that Schedule II drugs that must be kept refrigerated require their own locked refrigerator.

STORAGE OF COMPLETED PRESCRIPTIONS

For storage, completed prescriptions should be alphabetized by the name of the patient. If customers do not pick them up right away, they should be placed in a storage area or on shelves.

COMPUTER SYSTEMS

There are five major tasks in the pharmacy that a computerized system can handle efficiently:

- Prescription dispensing
- Record maintenance
- Clinical support
- Accounting
- Business management

Computer systems require special care and maintenance. The following factors may be damaging to computer systems:

- Dust
- Moisture
- Power surges
- Temperature
- Movement

EQUIPMENT FOR FILING, LABELING, AND PACKAGING

Computerized prescription information must be kept in the computer system, while hard copies must be kept in prescription files. There are various types of units available to store original prescription orders:

- Metal cabinets
- Cardboard containers
- Partitioned drawers
- Microfilm

Prescription labels can be created by a computer or a typewriter.

For packaging, there are various types of child-resistant caps for medication containers that hold tablets and capsules. For liquid medications, different sizes of bottles are available. For creams and ointments, appropriate jars, spatulas, and balances are required.

SINK

All pharmacy sinks must have hot and cold running water. These sinks must be used solely for purposes of disposal of expired medications. Eyewash facilities should be attached to the sink assembly because the risk of exposure to hazardous substances is prevalent in the pharmacy.

STORAGE FOR STOCK MEDICATIONS

Medications stored in bulk "stock bottles" are required to have the following information:

- Generic name
- Brand name
- Storage requirements:
  - Temperature (59° to 86° F)
  - Adequate ventilation
  - Air flow around the medication
  - Controlled humidity
  - Non-exposure to light
- Dosage form
- Quantity
- Controlled substance markings
- Expiration date
- Lot number

- Manufacturer's name
- National Drug Code (NDC) number

CONSULTATION AREA

Patient consultation *with the pharmacist* may sometimes be required.

The optimal setting for communication with a patient is a private consultation room adjacent to the dispensing area. The noise and distractions in a busy pharmacy can be handled using the following techniques:

- Move away from the pharmacy counter when possible to a more private area of the pharmacy.
- Ask other employees in the pharmacy not to interrupt during a patient session.
- Face the patient and speak clearly and distinctly in a tone loud enough to be heard, but not so loud as to be heard by others in the pharmacy.

Only the pharmacist is trained to consult with the patient. The pharmacy technician should refer patient questions related to their medications and therapies to the pharmacist.

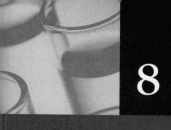

8

Hospital or Institutional Pharmacy

The practice of hospital pharmacy now encompasses all aspects of drug therapy, from the procurement of drugs and drug delivery devices, to their preparation, distribution, and most appropriate selection and use in each patient.

The operation and administration of hospital pharmacy varies from retail pharmacy. Technicians are an integral part of the pharmacy team, providing services such as procurement, storage, preparation, administration, and distribution of drugs and supplies to patients. Therefore, they must be familiar with all the aspects of, and their responsibilities in, the institutional pharmacy. ■

HOSPITAL PHARMACY

Hospital pharmacy is defined as the provision of pharmaceutical care within an institutional or hospital setting. The practice of pharmacy within institutional settings is completely different from that in community settings. Hospital pharmacy comprises four types of services:

1. Support services
2. Product services
3. Clinical services
4. Educational services

SUPPORT SERVICES

Support services include:

- Ordering and properly storing medications
- Maintaining an inventory of pharmaceuticals and medical supplies
- Billing for services
- Installing or maintaining computer systems

PRODUCT SERVICES

Product services deal with:

- Preparing, dispensing, and processing physicians' orders for inpatients
- Maintaining required patient and drug control records

CLINICAL SERVICES

Clinical services include:

- Managing the formulary system
- Evaluating drug use
- Reviewing drug orders for appropriateness

EDUCATIONAL SERVICES

Educational services deal with providing education about medications to pharmacy staff, other health-care professionals, the public, and patients and their caregivers.

ORGANIZATION OF THE HOSPITAL PHARMACY

The hospital pharmacy is the department responsible for all aspects of drug use. The pharmacy department includes personnel classified into three categories:

1. Professional—all pharmacists and management
2. Technical—pharmacy technicians involved in drug-related processes
3. Support—personnel involved in providing services that support drug-related processes and/or management functions

Larger hospital pharmacies may have many different positions and functions:

1. Management (pharmacists)
   a. Director
   b. Manager
   c. Supervisor
2. Dispensing and preparation
   a. Pharmacist
   b. Technician
   c. Central intravenous (IV) admixture and sterile processing may be done by both the pharmacist and technician, depending on state law.

    d. Controlled drug storage and distribution may also be handled by both the pharmacist and the technician, depending on state law.

3. Support (generally non-pharmacists)
    a. Department secretary
    b. Buyer
    c. Biller
    d. Systems analyst

4. Clinical
    a. Clinical coordinator
    b. Clinical pharmacist
    c. Clinical specialist

5. Education and research
    a. Drug-information specialist
    b. Research coordinator

Figure 8–1 demonstrates an organizational chart for the institutional pharmacy.

■ THE ROLES AND DUTIES OF PHARMACY TECHNICIANS IN HOSPITALS

The complexity of health care in the modern hospital has influenced revolutionary changes in the roles and duties of the pharmacy technicians who work in these settings. The job descriptions and responsibilities of these pharmacy technicians include:

- Ensure that policies and procedures are followed.
- Maintain medication records.
- Maintain competence in areas of responsibility.
- Prepare unit doses and floor stock medications.

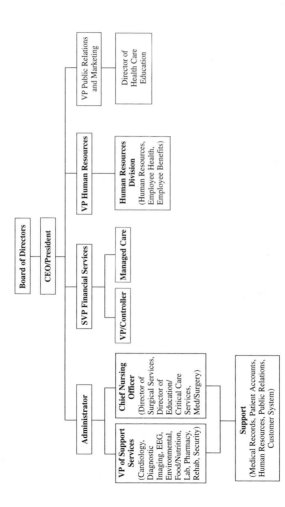

FIGURE 8–1 Sample of a hospital organizational chart.

- Utilize aseptic technique to prepare and mix intravenous, parenteral nutrition, and other admixtures.
- Package medications into unit-dose and unit-of-use packaging.
- Perform routine inspection of patient-care and medication-storage areas for medication control, security, and controlled-substance accountability.
- Prepare and deliver prescriptions to patients who are out of the hospital, such as those in nursing homes, hospice, and rehabilitation facilities.
- Maintain inventory.
- Order, receive, and restock medications.
- Prepare labels.
- Collect patient information to provide a complete medication profile.
- Input computer data.
- Maintain privacy.
- Possess and use communication skills.
- Use safe methods of working.
- Document medication preparation, packaging, and compounding.
- Enter charges and credits to ensure billing accuracy.
- Perform audits of medication processes.
- Complete controlled substance documentation.
- Avoid medication errors.

■ MEDICATION ORDERS

The practice of hospital pharmacy begins with the **medication order**, which is originated by the physician. The medication order, as used in hospital pharmacy, is the equivalent of the prescription in the retail pharmacy.

The medication order must contain the following information (see Figure 5–2; page 89):

- Patient's name, height, weight, medical condition, and known allergies
- Dosage schedule
- Instructions for preparing the drugs, based on the diagnosis and any patient allergies
- The exact dosage form of the drug
- The dosage strength
- Directions for use
- Route of administration

TYPES OF MEDICATION ORDERS

There are several types of medication orders, which include:

- ASAP orders
- Stat medication orders
- PRN (as needed) medication orders
- Emergency medication orders

- Controlled substance medication orders
- Scheduled medication orders
- Scheduled intravenous (IV)/total parenteral nutrition (TPN) solution orders
- Investigational medication orders

MEDICATION DISPENSING SYSTEMS

The number of prescriptions in the United States is rapidly increasing as the population grows older. This increase in prescriptions challenges the ability of available pharmacies and pharmacists to keep pace. The demand to process these prescriptions rapidly and accurately has influenced many administrators in purchasing robotic dispensing systems to make their operations more efficient, and to increase output possibilities in the pharmacy.

Prescription dispensing systems can fill and label up to 100 prescription vials per hour. Most robotic automation works with oral solids (for example, tablets and capsule) or ready-to-label products such as birth control pills.

THE FLOOR STOCK SYSTEM

In the **floor stock system**, the role of the pharmacy in the medication process is product related only. Pharmacy technicians are involved in repackaging these products. Drugs are purchased in bulk and multidose dosage forms. A medication could be used for more than one patient. The disadvantages of this system are as follows:

- Potential for medication errors
- Potential for drug diversion and misappropriation resulting in economic loss
- Increased inventory needs
- Inadequate space for medication storage on the patient care unit

THE UNIT-DOSE SYSTEM

The unit-dose system involves the preparation of medications in single-unit packages. It is considered to be the safest, most efficient, most effective medication system. Pharmacy technicians are also sometimes involved in repackaging drugs in this system. The features of the unit-dose system include:

- A copy of the original physician's order
- All medications are dispensed per individual patient.
- Individual doses of medications are labeled.
- More information must be provided, such as allergies and patient weight.
- No more than a 24-hour supply of medication is dispensed.

The advantages of using the unit-dose drug distribution system include:

- Improved medication control
- Reduction in medication errors
- Decreased overall cost of medication distribution
- More precise medication billing
- Reduction in medications returned unused
- Reduction in the size of drug inventories located in patient-care areas

Note: Most medications are commercially available in unit-dose form, but pharmacy technicians still must package other medications as unit-dose units. IV medications are the best examples of this type of packaging task. Many IV medications are not stable in solution and must be mixed by a technician just prior to administration.

PURCHASING SYSTEMS

The two types of purchasing systems include:

1. Independent purchasing
2. Group purchasing

INDEPENDENT PURCHASING

Independent purchasing means that pharmaceutical manufacturers may directly negotiate prices with the pharmacy buyers.

GROUP PURCHASING

Group purchasing involves the collaboration of many hospitals in negotiations with pharmaceutical manufacturers to achieve advantageous pricing and other benefits.

FORMS OF PURCHASING

There are several forms of purchasing:

1. Direct purchasing from the pharmaceutical manufacturer
2. Purchase from a wholesaler

3. Purchase from a prime vendor (the relationship between a hospital and a single wholesaler)
4. Purchase from a secondary vendor

Remember...

- Direct purchasing eliminates the middleman and handling fees, but requires a significant commitment of time, larger inventories, and more storage space.
- Purchasing from a wholesaler means that many items are purchased from one source.

ORDER PROCESSING

Information that must be processed when ordering includes the following:

- The name of the manufacturer
- The generic and brand name
- The strength and dosage form of the drug, or size of the device
- The quantity of drug dosage forms per package
- The type of packaging
- The number of bottles, packages, or devices being ordered

STORAGE OF MEDICATIONS

Medications and completed prescriptions should always be placed in a specific area or on shelves.

Prescriptions should be alphabetized by the name of the patient. Some of them require refrigeration; others should be kept away from light, or meet other storage requirements.

THE SHELF LIFE OF MEDICATIONS

Disposal requirements for most medications that have an expiration date are listed in package inserts or on material safety data sheets (MSDS). The shelf life of a medication is the time that it is allowed to be sold for use by patients. Expired drugs and how they are disposed of should be documented. They should be placed into containers labeled with "Expired Drugs—DO NOT USE" or a similar, clear warning. All expired, deteriorated, contaminated, or other nonreusable drug products must be removed immediately from usable pharmacy stock and disposed of.

MEDICATIONS NEEDING REFRIGERATION

Medications that require refrigeration must be kept in a pharmacy refrigerator solely used for the storage of drugs. No food or beverages are permitted to be stored in any refrigerator that contains medications. Temperatures must be kept between 2° and 8°C.

AUTOMATION

Significant progress has been made through the use of computers and hardware technologies such as automation devices, robots, and point-of-care automated dispensing technology. Automation provides the ability to rapidly process large volumes of medication orders accurately and quickly.

QUALITY CONTROL

Quality control is a process of checks and balances followed during the manufacturing of a product or provision of a service to ensure that the end products exceed specified standards such as zero problems or zero errors.

COMPOUNDING MEDICATIONS

Compounding is the preparation, mixing, assembling, packaging, and labeling of a drug product based on a prescription order from a licensed practitioner for an individual patient. Compounding drugs may be classified as non-sterile and sterile compounding (parenteral and intravenous admixture) drugs and will be discussed in Chapters 10 and 11.

■ INVENTORY MANAGEMENT

There are six types of inventory management:

1. *Order book system*—This system relies on the person dispensing a product to determine whether a product needs to be reordered.

2. *Inventory record card system*—This system relies on the maintenance of an ongoing use and purchase history on a card or paper system.

3. *ABC inventory system*—This system is more sophisticated, and is not widely employed by many institutional pharmacies.

4. *Economic order quantity (EOQ) and economic order value (EOV) system*—These are the same as the ABC inventory system.

5. *Computerized inventory system*—This system is evolving as automation and technology expand; it eliminates ongoing personnel needs for inventory management.

6. *Minimum/maximum level system*—This system relies on a predetermined order point and order quantity, which are based on historical use.

Note: Most hospital pharmacies use the order book system or the computerized inventory system.

INVENTORY TURNOVER RATE

The **inventory turnover rate** can determine the effectiveness of the inventory-control system. This is a mathematical calculation of the number of times the average inventory is replaced over a period of time (annually):

$$\text{Inventory turnover rate} = \frac{\text{Purchases for period}}{\text{Average inventory for period}}$$

$$\text{Average Inventory} = \frac{\text{Beginning inventory for period} + \text{Ending inventory for period}}{2}$$

SAFETY

A safe working environment in the institutional pharmacy must always be maintained to ensure the health and safety of pharmacy personnel. Work areas must be clean. Accidental exposures to harmful substances must be avoided. Emergency and exposure treatment plans must be in place. Pharmacy technicians must be aware of unsafe conditions and be able to quickly respond to them.

THE POLICY AND PROCEDURE MANUAL

The complexity of the hospital organization requires that the hospital and all its departments must have a set of standard operating statements to operate effectively and efficiently. In support of the hospital and health-care delivery system, the pharmacy department must develop guidelines for operations. This document is formally called the Policy and Procedure Manual. It should answer the following questions:

- What action must be undertaken?
- What is its purpose?
- When must it be done?
- Where must it be done?
- Who should do it?
- How must it be done?

REGULATORY AGENCIES THAT OVERSEE HOSPITAL PHARMACY

The following agencies oversee all aspects of hospital operations:

- The Joint Commission

- State Board of Pharmacy (BOP)
- Centers for Medicare and Medicaid Services (CMS)
- Department of Public Health (DPH)

THE JOINT COMMISSION

The **Joint Commission** is an independent, voluntary agency that surveys and accredits health-care organizations. Joint Commission standards of practice for pharmacies include:

- Preparing a comprehensive operations manual
- Clearly defined areas of responsibility and lines of authority
- Written job descriptions that are developed and revised as required
- Manual revisions, including continuing changes
- Familiarization of all institutional personnel with the manual's contents
- Obtaining input from other medical disciplines

CMS

Another important agency that affects institutional pharmacy operations is the **Centers for Medicare/Medicaid Services**, which administers the Medicare, Medicaid, and Child Health Insurance Programs, providing health insurance for over 74 million people in the United States. It also regulates all laboratory testing in the United States (except research). This agency inspects and approves hospitals to provide care for Medicaid patients. The CMS must approve covered patients in order for them to receive reimbursement.

STATE BOARD OF PHARMACY

The **State Board of Pharmacy (BOP)** is an agency that registers pharmacists as well as pharmacy technicians. Twenty-two states require that pharmacy technicians be certified or registered.

DEPARTMENT OF PUBLIC HEALTH

The **Department of Public Health (DPH)** oversees and inspects hospitals, including their pharmacies, to assure compliance with laws concerning hospital practice.

9

Advanced Pharmacy

Pharmacy practice has expanded over the years into non-traditional areas such as mail-order, home infusion, hospice, ambulatory care, nuclear, long-term, and compounding pharmacies. The primary goal is to reduce health-care costs and increase the overall quality of life for the patient. Pharmacy technicians must be trained, skillful, and knowledgeable in these areas. Pharmacy technicians work under the direct supervision of a pharmacist. ■

▌MAIL-ORDER PHARMACY

A **mail-order pharmacy** is a type of pharmacy that dispenses maintenance medications to members through mail delivery. A maintenance medication is a drug that is taken on an ongoing basis for a chronic condition, such as:

- Diabetes
- High blood pressure
- High cholesterol
- Asthma

- Arthritis
- Depression
- Gastrointestinal disorders

Mail-order pharmacies provide services to all 50 states, and they must follow federal and state requirements in processing prescriptions.

ADVANTAGES

The advantages of a mail-order pharmacy include:

- Cost savings
- Patient convenience
- Improved compliance
- Improved pharmacy efficiency
- Decreased dispensing errors
- Patient privacy
- Availability of medications

DISADVANTAGES

- Lack of personal contact
- Limited access to a pharmacist
- Medication waste
- Time delays

STAFF MEMBERS

Staff members of mail-order pharmacies consist of:

- Licensed pharmacists
- Pharmacy technicians
- Registered nurses

THE ROLE OF PHARMACY TECHNICIANS

Pharmacy technicians must be specially trained to work in mail-order pharmacies. Because mail-order pharmacies are highly automated, each technician can be responsible for different steps in the prescription process. The following are examples of the roles of technicians in mail-order pharmacies:

- Entering prescriptions into the system
- Dispensing prescriptions
- Preparing prescriptions for shipping

Remember...

Steps must be taken by the pharmacist in checking and reviewing the prescription before and after filling the prescription.

INTERNET PHARMACY

Internet pharmacies are revolutionizing the prescription drug market. They are also referred to as online pharmacies. These pharmacies run much like mail-order pharmacies. Some Internet pharmacies offer personal contact between pharmacists and patients via e-mail. Two of the best-known Internet pharmacies are:

- http://www.cvs.com
- http://www.drugstore.com

Internet pharmacy is also known as:

- e pharmacy
- Online pharmacy
- Cyberpharmacy

Internet pharmacy consists of three types:

- Those involved in providing legend pharmaceuticals pursuant to a valid prescription order
- Those that offer free information and counseling but do not dispense medications
- Those that interact with medical professionals, government personnel, regulatory agencies, and also society at large

Important points to remember about Internet pharmacy include:

- Buying drugs online may put one's health at serious risk.
- A health-care practitioner should examine the customer in person before the customer buys drugs online.
- Ensure that the Internet pharmacy offers a street address and telephone number, as well as a way of contacting its pharmacist(s).
- Prescription drugs should be purchased from an Internet pharmacy only by prescription. Beware of online pharmacies that offer prescription medications without a prescription, or that offer to issue a prescription based on answers to an online questionnaire.
- Do not buy prescription drugs from an Internet pharmacy that claims to have a "miracle cure" for any serious condition.

- The Internet pharmacy should always have the drug's I.D. number listed.
- Contact the Better Business Bureau (http://www.bbb.org) about any Internet pharmacy whose legitimacy is questionable before purchasing anything from the pharmacy.

ADVANTAGES

Internet pharmacies are being recognized as:

- Convenient
- Easy-to-use
- Cost-effective
- Providers of prescription and nonprescription medications
- Providers of vitamins, herbals, and health and beauty products
- Able to accept patients' prescription drug insurance and charge the co-pay to a credit card account
- Delivering promptly (overnight)
- Providers of toll-free telephone lines or e-mail addresses that offer information on medications and diseases
- High-volume dispensing operations
- Having extensive safeguards
- Having secure Websites
- Being licensed in all states

DISADVANTAGES

The disadvantages of Internet pharmacies often become apparent only after a purchase has been made. Some of these disadvantages include:

- Fake, outdated, or unapproved products
- Little or no quality control
- Possibility of incorrect diagnoses
- Dispensing of inappropriate medicines
- Lack of confidentiality and/or security

STAFF MEMBERS

The staff members of reputable Internet pharmacies may include any of the following, depending on the complete range of services provided:

- Licensed pharmacists
- Pharmacy technicians
- Registered nurses
- Registered respiratory therapists
- Sales and marketing professionals
- Administrative staff with customer service experience

THE ROLE OF PHARMACY TECHNICIANS

Pharmacy technicians working in an online pharmacy assist the pharmacists and other pharmacy staff in a variety of ways, including:

- Receiving order requests for prescriptions from patients
- Recording information in the computer system
- Dispensing medications

- Packaging medications for shipment
- Answering questions from patients that do not require a pharmacist's answer

VERIFIED INTERNET PHARMACY PRACTICE SITES (VIPPS)

The VIPPS program was launched by the National Association of Boards of Pharmacy to approve and identify online pharmacies that are appropriately licensed and prepared to practice Internet pharmacy. Any online pharmacy seeking VIPPS certification must:

- Secure pharmacy licensure from the board of pharmacy in each state into which it ships pharmaceuticals
- Undergo an on-site review by a VIPPS inspection team
- Submit written policies and procedures to NAPB that assure compliance with VIPPS criteria
- Meet a stringent 17-point set of criteria, including:
  - Verification of appropriate licensure in each state in which the pharmacy does business
  - Establishment of appropriate patient privacy, authentication, and security measures
  - Maintenance of a quality-assurance program
  - Establishment of meaningful, appropriate consultations between pharmacists and patients
  - Establishment of procedures to contact prescribers or patients if a delay occurs in the delivery of pharmaceuticals
  - Provision of a method of informing caregivers and patients of drug recalls

- Provision of an education program for both patients and caregivers about the appropriate means of disposal of expired or unusable medications

Remember...

Once an online pharmacy becomes VIPPS certified, the NAPB continues to monitor the pharmacy. This includes annual reviews, recertifications, and follow-up site inspections.

HOME INFUSION PHARMACY

A home infusion pharmacy is defined as a pharmacy that prepares and dispenses infusion therapies to patients in the home and alternative sites. There are many types of infusion therapies prescribed by physicians that are suitable for home infusion. These infusion therapies include:

- Intravenous (IV) solutions
- Other injectable drugs
- Enteral nutrition therapy
- Total parenteral nutrition (TPN)
- Pain-management therapy
- Anti-infective therapy
- Hydration therapy
- Chemotherapy
- Biotechnology therapy (genetic engineering)
- Miscellaneous therapies such as heparin, diuretics, steroids, and H_2-receptor antagonists

ADVANTAGES

Home infusion pharmacies offer:

- The freedom for patients to recover in their own home
- The opportunity for patients to participate in their care plan
- Better cost-effectiveness for most insurance companies

DISADVANTAGES

Home infusion pharmacies do not offer:

- Interaction with customers
- Interaction with third-party plans

STAFF MEMBERS

The staff of a home infusion pharmacy consists of:

- Licensed pharmacists
- Registered nurses
- Pharmacy technicians

THE ROLE OF PHARMACY TECHNICIANS

Pharmacy technicians may be involved in the compounding of sterile products and the handling of home infusion equipment and supplies. The pharmacy technician must possess traditional pharmacy knowledge and skills as well as knowledge and skills specific to home infusion pharmacy, such as:

- Knowledge of the home infusion process
- Complete knowledge of sterile compounding
- Excellent aseptic technique

- Knowledge of and skill in handling pharmaceutical calculations
- Familiarity with home infusion equipment and supplies
- Knowledge of documenting and record keeping in home infusion pharmacy
- Excellent computer skills
- Familiarity with legislation and regulations

■ HOSPICE PHARMACY

The purpose of a hospice pharmacy is to provide medications and pharmaceutical care to the hospice patient to enhance the quality of his or her remaining life. Hospice patients are terminally ill with one or more of the following diagnoses:

- Cancer
- AIDS
- Alzheimer's disease
- Congestive heart failure
- Other terminal illnesses

The only element that differentiates a hospice pharmacy from other areas of pharmacy is its inventory. The inventory in a hospice pharmacy is limited and specialized. It does not include all of the medications used for the treatment of diseases. The hospice pharmacy stock includes more types of dosage forms of medication, such as injectables and suppositories, for terminally ill patients who cannot take oral medications. Examples of these drugs include:

- Narcotic and non-narcotic analgesics
- Anti-nauseants
- Laxatives
- Antianxiety medications
- IV infusions for pain therapy, hydration therapy, etc.

ADVANTAGES

Hospice pharmacy offers the following advantages:

- One-on-one, comforting patient care treating the person, not the disease
- Emphasis on quality of the remaining life of the patient
- Twenty-four-hour help and support
- Follow-up with the patient's family after the patient's death

DISADVANTAGES

The disadvantages of hospice pharmacy include:

- Limitations exist concerning what Medicare covers for hospice patients.
- Money is wasted on medications that are left unused after a patient's death, and which, by law, cannot be repackaged for use by others.

STAFF MEMBERS

The staff of a hospice pharmacy includes:

- Licensed and specialized pharmacists
- Pharmacy technicians

- Administrative personnel
- Drivers who deliver medications

THE ROLE OF PHARMACY TECHNICIANS

Pharmacy technicians in hospice pharmacy are responsible for:

- Filling and packaging prescriptions intended to provide utmost patient comfort, including intravenous therapies
- Providing pain- and symptom-management information
- Providing drug information and education

NUCLEAR PHARMACY

Nuclear pharmacy is possibly the most specialized practice setting for pharmacists and pharmacy technicians. It involves handling radioactive materials, and it involves some unique sterile compounding. To work in nuclear pharmacy, technicians must carry the following qualifications:

- Special knowledge
- Special training
- Skill in sterile compounding
- Familiarity with radiation safety
- Familiarity with specific legislation and regulations that pertain to nuclear pharmacy practice

RADIOACTIVE DRUGS

Radiopharmaceuticals are used for diagnosing and treating disease. The majority of them, about 90 percent, are used for diagnosis. Radioactive drugs release radiation within the body. They are available in many dosage forms, such as:

- Oral capsules ("seeds")
- Pellets (for implanting into the body)
- Oral solutions
- Sterile injections
- Sterile gases

Radioactive drugs usually consist of two parts:

- Radionuclides
- Carrier drugs

Examples of carrier drugs and their sites of action are listed in Table 9–1.

TABLE 9–1 Most Common Carrier Drugs

Carrier Drug	Site of Action
Cardiolyte (sestamibi)	Heart
Choletec (mebrofenin)	Liver
MAA (microaggregated albumin)	Lungs
MDP (medronate)	Bones
Techniscan (mertiatide or MAG_3)	Kidneys

The most common radioactive drugs that are used for diagnosis are listed in Table 9–2.

TABLE 9–2 Most Common Radioactive Drugs for Diagnosis

Radiopharmaceutical	Indications
^{99m}Tc-MAA	Lung perfusion study
^{99m}Tc-MDP	Bone and skeletal imaging
^{99m}Tc-mebrofenin	Liver imaging
^{99m}Tc-sestamibi	Heart perfusion study
^{99m}Tc-MAG3	Kidney function

INVENTORY

A separate class of drugs is used in the nuclear pharmacy. Radioactive drugs have short half-lives, usually several hours, and lose a substantial amount of their radioactivity if stored for any period of time. Therefore, radionuclides are ordered daily and only in the amounts that are needed.

PHARMACY DESIGN

The design of a nuclear pharmacy must:

- Protect the personnel from radiation exposure
- Prevent radioactive contamination of the pharmacy work area and equipment
- Ensure proper ventilation of the pharmacy
- Provide for the safe disposal of radioactive waste

- Limit access into the pharmacy
- Ensure the security of the pharmacy

The nuclear pharmacy is divided into different areas designed to handle specific tasks. They include:

- Breakdown area
- Order-entry area
- Compounding area (dispensing area)
- Quality-control area
- Packaging area
- Storage and disposal area

EQUIPMENT AND SUPPLIES

There is quite a wide variety of specialized equipment found in the nuclear pharmacy. This equipment includes:

- Laminar airflow hood
- Glove box
- Dose calibrator
- Dosimeter
- Lead-lined refrigerator and freezer
- Lead-lined storage boxes
- Autoclave
- Heating equipment
- Testing equipment
- Lead barrier shield
- Deep stainless steel sink
- Shower

Figures 9–1, 9–2, 9–3, and 9–4 are examples of nuclear pharmacy.

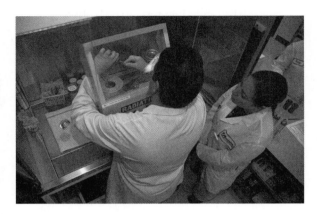

FIGURE 9–1   **Nuclear pharmacy is another area of specialization for pharmacy technicians.**

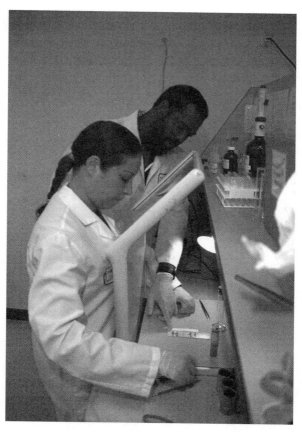

FIGURE 9–2 One of the primary duties within nuclear pharmacy is that of compounding radiopharmaceuticals.

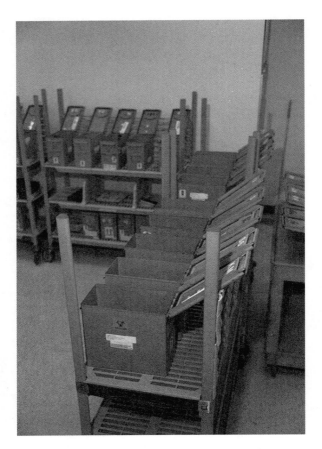

FIGURE 9–3 Special precautions must be taken in the handling, care, storage, and distribution of radioactive materials.

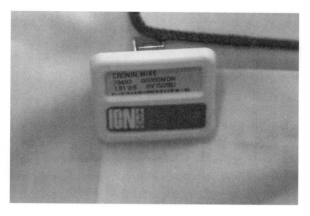

FIGURE 9–4   Staff within the nuclear pharmacy must wear devices to monitor the amount of radiation exposure they experience while on the job.

NUCLEAR PHARMACY ADVANTAGES

- Specialized products that are vital for treating specific conditions
- Delivery of radiopharmaceuticals

NUCLEAR PHARMACY DISADVANTAGES

- Short shelf life of radioactive products
- Busy staff due to demands of many medical facilities needing their services
- Possible exposure to hazardous radioactive materials

STAFF MEMBERS

The nuclear pharmacy staff usually consists of:

- Licensed and specialized nuclear pharmacists
- Specially trained pharmacy technicians
- Administrative staff members
- Drivers

THE ROLE OF PHARMACY TECHNICIANS

Nuclear pharmacy technicians are required to:

- Prepare the patient- and organ-specific doses and accurately label all radiopharmaceuticals
- Unpack lead-encased "generators" containing radioactive parent material
- "Wipe" off the generators to document their level of radioactivity
- Perform quality-control testing
- Calibrate equipment

◼ LONG-TERM-CARE PHARMACY

Long-term-care pharmacy is the primary source of medications for long-term care or nursing home residents. A long-term-care pharmacy can be found in a variety of styles and settings. The long-term-care pharmacy provides various services to the long-term-care facility to ensure the following:

- Safe ordering
- Distribution
- Storage

- Administration
- Accountability
- Record keeping of medications

DRUG-DISTRIBUTION SYSTEMS

A drug-distribution system is a safe and economical method for the distribution of a drug. It refers to the packaging or container that holds and stores the drug during its transfer from the pharmacy to the patient. A pharmacy technician should become familiar with various drug-distribution systems available for use in the long-term-care setting, such as:

- Unit-dose system
- Modified unit-dose system
- Traditional vial system
- Automated dispensing systems
- Specialized medication dispensers

EMERGENCY MEDICATION SUPPLY

An emergency supply of medications in limited quantities is kept in long-term-care facilities. Emergency drugs to be kept in a long-term care facility are determined by the:

- Long-term-care pharmacist
- Representatives from the medical nursing staff
- State regulations

Medication categories in the emergency medication supply include:

- Analgesics
- Antibiotics

- Anticoagulants and vitamin K
- Antidiarrheals
- Antidysrhythmics
- Antihistamines
- Antinauseants
- Antipsychotics
- Diuretics
- Hyperglycemics and hypoglycemics
- IV additives
- Large-volume parenterals
- Narcotic antagonists
- Poison-control medications
- Seizure-control medications

ADVANTAGES

Long-term-care pharmacy offers:

- Twenty-four-hour service
- Delivery of medications to nursing facilities
- Special packaging that aids in safe administration of medications
- Emergency supply of medications kept on hand
- Frequent safety reviews of pharmacy services
- All long-term-care facility residents served regardless of financial situation

DISADVANTAGES

Long-term-care pharmacies are generally excellent, with no clearly identifiable disadvantages.

STAFF MEMBERS

The staff of a long-term-care pharmacy may include:

- Licensed and specialized pharmacists
- Pharmacy technicians
- Administration personnel
- Drivers who deliver medications

THE ROLE OF PHARMACY TECHNICIANS

The role of pharmacy technicians in long-term-care pharmacies may include:

- Data collecting and reporting
- Surveys and inspections
- Education
- Maintenance
- Dispensing
- Inventory

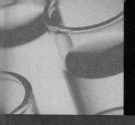

10

Nonsterile Compounding

Compounding of drugs might be one of the duties of the pharmacy technician. Pharmaceutical compounding requires that technicians use their training in mathematics, science, and technology more often than some of the other practices of pharmacy. Compounding of a drug includes:

- The Food and Drug Administration (FDA)
- Preparation
- Mixing
- Assembling
- Packaging
- Labeling

Pharmacy technicians must be familiar with compounding procedures (for sterile and nonsterile medications) and equipment. Technicians also must receive proper orientation before being given this responsibility.

For compounding medications, pharmacists must comply with laws, regulations, and standards that govern the preparation of compounded products. Compliance relates to all of the following:

- Organization and personnel
- Drug-compounding facilities
- Proper materials
- Equipment
- Drug product containers and closures
- Drug-compounding controls
- Dispensing
- Labeling
- Storage
- Documented techniques ▪

EQUIPMENT

Correct equipment is important when compounding. Many state boards of pharmacy have a required minimum list of equipment for compounding medications. Technicians must be familiar with all equipment that will be used. The most conventional pieces of equipment and instruments that you may use are as follows:

- Balances (Class A prescription balance and/or electronic scale)
- Weights
- Spatulas
- Compounding slabs
- Hot plates
- Mortars
- Pestles
- Beakers
- Tongs
- Heat guns
- Graduates
- Pipettes
- Compounding logbook

BALANCES

Balances are pieces of equipment that may be used for weighing. There are two types: a **class A prescription balance** (an electronic scale) and a **counter balance**. Class A prescription balances are used for weighing small amounts of drugs that are not more than 120 grams (see Figure 10–1).

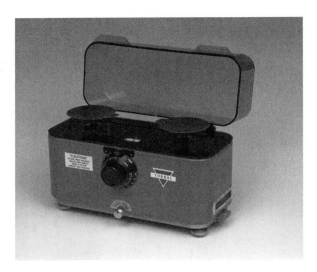

FIGURE 10–1 **Class A prescription balance.**

Remember...

Electronic scales are used more often than torsion balances.

A counter balance is capable of weighing larger quantities, up to about 5 kilograms. A counter balance is not used for prescription compounding. It is used for measuring bulk quantities.

WEIGHTS

Weights made from corrosion-resistant metals, such as brass, are preferred (see Figure 10–2). In Figure 10–2, metric weights are in the front row and Apothecary weights are in the back row.

SPATULAS

Spatulas are used to transfer solid and semi-solid ingredients such as powders, creams, and ointments to weighing pans. They are also used to mix compounds on an ointment slab (see Figure 10–3).

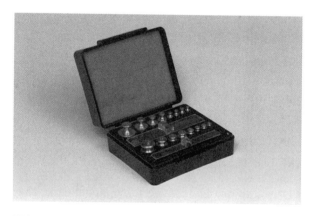

FIGURE 10–2   Weights used in pharmaceutical practice.

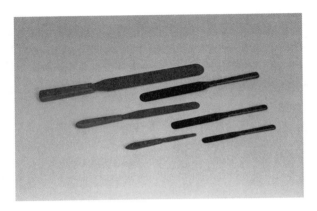

FIGURE 10–3   Spatulas.

COMPOUNDING SLABS

Compounding slabs are plates made of ground glass with hard, flat, and nonabsorbent surfaces that are ideal for mixing compounds (see Figure 10–4).

HOT PLATES

Hot plates, heated iron plates, are used to heat substances (usually adjustable between 50 and 300 degrees Celsius) as may be required for compounding. They are available in various sizes with various features. Some laboratory-grade hot plates offer an attached

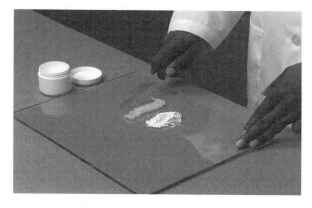

FIGURE 10–4   Compounding slab.

contact thermometer, and coated surfaces that resist impact, scratches, and acids.

MORTARS

A **mortar** is a cup-shaped vessel in which materials are ground or crushed by a pestle in the preparation of drugs.

PESTLES

A **pestle** is a mixing tool often used in the preparation of a compounded prescription. It is normally used along with a mortar (see Figure 10–5).

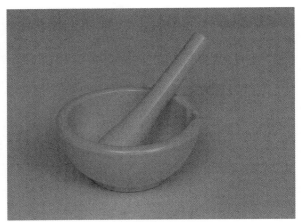

A

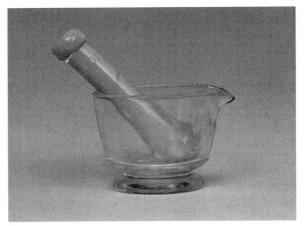

B

FIGURE 10–5 (A) Porcelain mortar and pestle.
(B) Glass mortar and pestle.

BEAKERS

A **beaker** is a type of equipment used to heat substances for compounding. Beakers are made of various materials, such as:

- Glass
- Stainless steel
- Plastic

Beakers come in various sizes (50, 100, 150, 250, 400, 600, 1000 mL) and are often coated with cork to protect the person handling the beaker.

TONGS

Tongs are devices used for handling hot beakers. They are similar in design to tongs used to pick up ice cubes, but generally are sized for the specific task of working with beakers. They are usually made of nickel, stainless steel, or polystyrene and are available in a variety of designs, including some with protective coatings to protect users from burns.

HEAT GUNS

Heat guns are basically the same devices as hand-held hair dryers, but in pharmacy are instruments used for melting and polishing:

- Suppositories
- Lozenges
- Troches

GRADUATES

Pharmaceutical liquids are measured in glass or plastic **graduates** of various sizes and shapes. There are two types: conical and cylindrical graduates. Conical graduates are easier to handle and clean. Cylindrical graduates are designed with a narrow diameter that is the same from top to base. Cylindrical forms are more accurate than conical graduates. Both types are generally calibrated in metric units (cubic centimeters), and conical graduates are mostly calibrated in both metric and apothecary units (see Figure 10–6 and Figure 10–7).

Remember...

To accurately read a graduate scale, one must read the level at the bottom of the meniscus (a concave surface that looks like a double line) while holding the graduate at eye level.

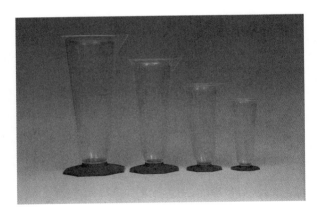

FIGURE 10–6   Conical graduates.

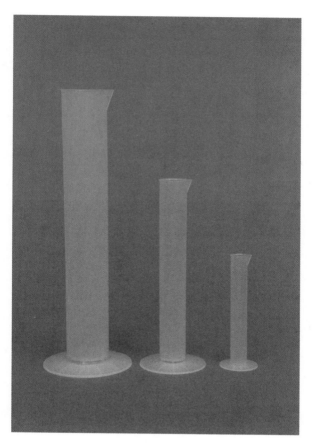

FIGURE 10–7   Cylindrical graduates.

PIPETTES

A **pipette** can be used for measurement of volumes of liquids less than 1.5 mL. Pipettes are long, cylindrical, calibrated tubes that are used to deliver or transfer specified volumes of liquid. Drawing liquids into the pipette requires a bulb or a vacuum pump-type device.

Remember...

Mouth-pipetting is forbidden.

■ COMPOUNDED PREPARATIONS

Compounded preparations are medications that have been prepared using more than one component. Sometimes commercially available dosage forms are not suitable for certain patients. Compounding is a method of customizing medications for individual patients and their needs. In manufactured medications, there is no specific patient in mind when the medication is produced. Patients are matched to the drugs that are available. Economic considerations limit available choices in drug dosages and dosage forms. Compounded medications offer the administration of a drug to the site of action in the most effective dosage form available.

■ COMPOUNDING PROCESSES

Preventing medication errors is the goal of the compounding process. Technicians must observe the following guidelines in the compounding process:

- Evaluate the appropriateness of the prescription.
- Accurately calculate the amount of ingredients.
- Determine proper equipment needed.

- Follow handwashing, gloving, and gowning procedures.
- Evaluate the final medication for weight variations and proper mixing.
- Make proper notes in the compounding log.
- Use appropriate labeling.

COMPOUNDING RECORDS AND DOCUMENTS

In the pharmacy, record keeping and documentation is essential, particularly for compounding drugs. The compounding record is the log or record of an actual batch of medication being prepared. It includes:

- Manufacturer names of chemicals used
- The date of preparation
- Lot numbers of chemicals used
- Expiration date
- Chemicals in the formula
- Equipment needed to prepare the formula
- Mixing instructions for preparing the formula

Compounding medications requires complete record keeping for the following reasons:

- Tracking chemicals
- Tracking the building of formulas from the chemicals
- Batching formula preparation into logs

There are two types of record keeping:

- Manual, with formulas and logs of individual lots kept on paper
- Using software and computers for tracking each step

■ COMMONLY COMPOUNDED PRODUCTS

Commonly compounded products include:

- Solutions
- Suspensions
- Suppositories
- Capsules
- Tablets
- Powders
- Transdermal or topical preparations (less commonly compounded than those previously listed)

COMPOUNDING SOLUTIONS

A **solution** is a liquid dosage form in which active ingredients are dissolved in a liquid vehicle. Liquid compounds are the most commonly compounded type of preparations in the pharmacy. There are two types of solutions: sterile and nonsterile compounding solutions. Sterile compounding solutions include sterile parenteral and ophthalmic solutions (these are discussed in Chapter 11). Nonsterile solutions are oral and topical solutions. The following are a few examples of oral liquid solutions:

- Syrups
- Elixirs
- Aromatic waters

COMPOUNDING SUSPENSIONS

A **suspension** is a liquid dosage form that contains solid drug particles dispersed in a liquid medium.

Solutions and suspensions may be oil-based, but are more commonly water-based. Dosing can be individualized to the patient by varying the concentration of the medication.

Compounding Equipment for Solutions and Suspensions

The following equipment is required for the compounding of solutions or suspensions:

- Mortars
- Pestles
- Light-resistant containers
- Auxiliary labels
- Suspending vehicles, such as:
  - Carboxymethylcellulose
  - Methylcellulose
  - Bentonite
  - Tragacanth
- Solid drugs
- Refrigerators

Procedure for Compounding Suspensions

Procedures for compounding suspensions include:

- The particle size is reduced by using a mortar and pestle to grind tablets or powders (Figure 10–8).
- This grounded powder must be moistened with an agent such as alcohol or glycerin, still using the mortar and pestle (Figure 10–9).
- The moistening agent is added in portions.
- Mixing with the mortar and pestle is continued until a uniform mixture results.

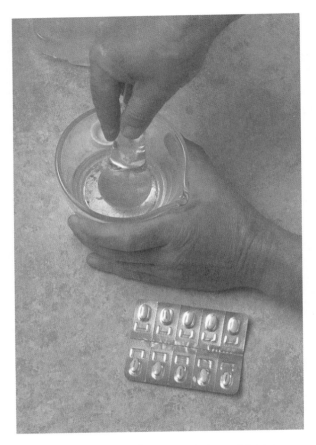

FIGURE 10–8   The technician grinds a tablet into a powder.

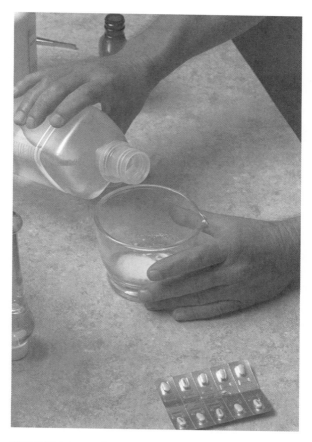

FIGURE 10–9 The technician adds solution to the powder.

- The remaining vehicle is blended with the mixture.
- The mortar and pestle can be rinsed with small portions of the vehicle so that all of the powdered agent is mixed with the moistened agent, until the final desired volume is reached.
- The suspension is dispensed in a tight, light-resistant container (Figure 10–10).
- The auxiliary label "Shake well" must be attached to the suspension container (Figure 10–11).

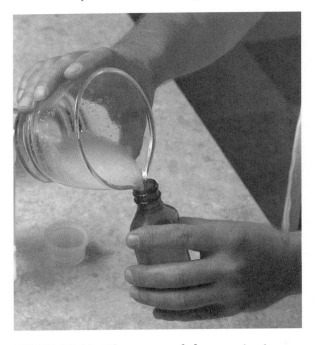

FIGURE 10–10 **The compounded suspension is poured into the patient's bottle.**

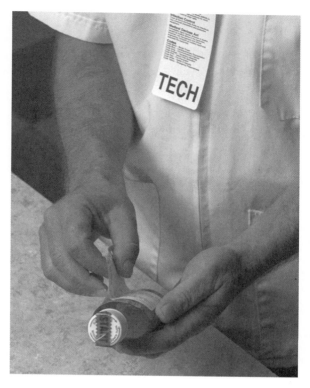

FIGURE 10–11   The technician labels the bottle.

COMPOUNDING SUPPOSITORIES

Suppositories are solid bodies of various weights and shapes, adapted for introduction into the rectum, vagina, or urethra. They are used to deliver drugs for local or systemic effects. There are three common suppository bases:

1. Cocoa butter (theobroma oil)
2. Polyethylene glycol (Carbowax)
3. Glycerinated gelatin

Suppositories are made using molds. The molds are made of brass, aluminum, rubber, or disposable plastic.

Compounding Equipment for Suppositories

The equipment required for compounding suppositories includes:

- Hot plates
- Mixing tools
- Molds
- Special boxes
- Labels
- Refrigerator

Procedure for Compounding Suppositories

Suppositories are prepared by:

1. Melting the base (Figure 10–12). Care must be taken to monitor the temperature to prevent overheating. Overheating the base may prevent it from returning to a solid form.
2. Incorporating the medications uniformly into the base (Figure 10–13).
3. Pouring the mixture into the suppository mold (Figure 10–14).

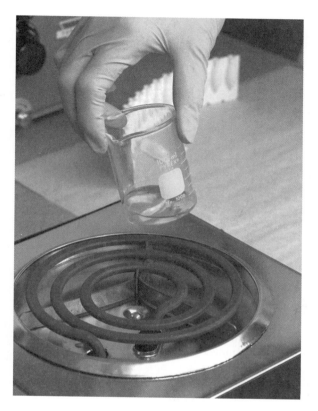

**FIGURE 10–12   The technician melts the base
material that will be combined with the powder.**

4. Dispensing in special boxes.
5. Labeling the container.
6. Storage (refrigerated).
7. Instructing the patient to store the suppositories
   in a cool, dry place.

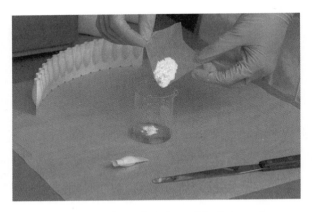

FIGURE 10–13   **The technician adds the powder to the melted base material.**

COMPOUNDING CAPSULES

Capsules are solid dosage forms in which the drug is enclosed within either a hard or soft soluble container or shell. The shells are usually made from a suitable gelatin. Hard gelatin capsules may be manually filled for extemporaneous compounding. There are numerous capsule sizes and colors. In the past, capsules were packed by hand, but now, capsule-filling machines are commonly used.

Capsule sizes range from number 5, the smallest, to number 000, the largest. Number 000 is usually the largest size used for patients.

Compounding Equipment for Capsules

The equipment used for compounding capsules includes:

- Mortars
- Pestles

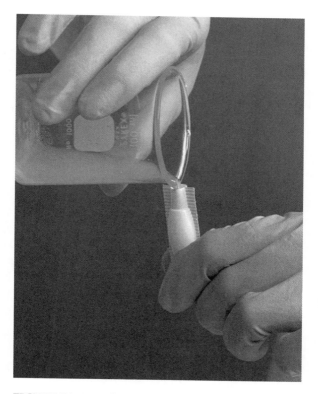

FIGURE 10–14 The technician pours the mixture into the suppository mold.

- Spatulas
- Pill tiles
- Active ingredients
- Bulk powders

- Scales
- Storage containers

Procedure for Compounding Capsules

Capsules are prepared by the following steps:

1. The bulk powders and all ingredients are triturated and blended using geometric dilution.
2. The appropriate size empty capsule is chosen.
3. The body and cap of the capsule are separated.
4. The powder formulation is compressed with a spatula on a pill tile.
5. The empty capsule body is filled with the powder until full (Figure 10–15).
6. The capsule is weighed to ensure an accurate dose.
7. The capsule is dispensed in a suitable container (Figure 10–16).
8. The product is stored.

COMPOUNDING TABLETS

Tablets are solid dosage forms containing medicinal substances with or without suitable diluents. They may vary in shape, size, and weight. Tablets may be classed according to the method of manufacture, such as molded tablets and compressed tablets.

Compounding Equipment for Tablets

The equipment used for compounding tablets includes:

- Molds
- Glass slabs

- Mixing containers
- Powders
- Alcohol or distilled water
- Mixing tools

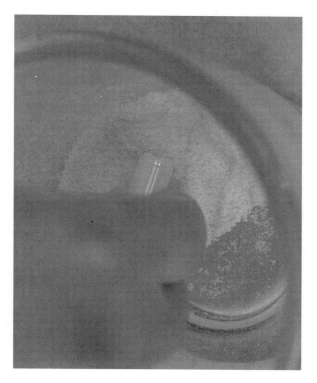

FIGURE 10–15   The technician "punches" the powdered mixture into the empty capsule shell.

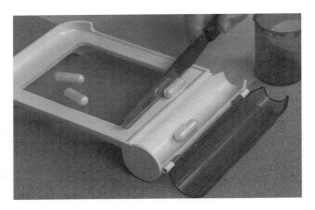

FIGURE 10–16 The technician counts the compounded capsules for dispensing.

- Drying pegs
- Storage containers

Procedure for Compounding Tablets

Tablets are prepared by the following steps:

1. Moisten the powder mixture with alcohol and water.
2. Add to a diluent, a mixture of lactose and sucrose (80/20), and a moistening agent.
3. Make a mixture of ethyl alcohol and water (60/40).
4. Dilute the mixture with the active ingredients.
5. Make a paste by using the alcohol and water mixture.
6. Mix and spread the paste into the mold.

7. Punch out the tablets and dry them on pegs.
8. Dispense the tablets once they are dried.

COMPOUNDING POWDERS

Powders are the finely ground form of an active drug. Powdered drugs are available in different forms, which include:

- Capsules
- Reconstituted with sterile water before being packaged in glass vials
- Packets (reconstituted with water for oral use)
- Sprinkled on topically, or sprayed on
- Inhaled into the lungs with an inhalation device

Compounding Equipment for Powders

Equipment for compounding powders includes:

- Pulverizing tools
- Scales
- Powder papers
- Powder boxes

Procedure for Compounding Powders

Preparation of powders depends on the route of administration used: internally or topically. The following steps should be taken:

1. Pulverize and blend the bulk powder.
2. Weigh each dose individually.
3. Transfer onto a powder paper and fold the paper.
4. Dispense the folded papers in a powder box.

COMPOUNDING TRANSDERMAL, OR TOPICAL DOSAGE, FORM DRUGS

Transdermal, or topical, medications are absorbed slowly through the skin, creating a constant, time-released systemic effect. Transdermal patches adhere to the skin and release very small amounts of the drug at a constant rate, carried from the skin by the capillaries. Common transdermal drugs include: estrogen, nicotine, nitroglycerin, scopolamine, testosterone, and formulas to relieve pain.

Drugs that may be applied topically to the skin or mucous membranes are semisolid dosage forms, and include ointments, creams, pastes, and gels. Ointments are characterized as being oily. Creams are generally oil-in-water emulsions. Pastes are characterized by their high content of solids. Gels consist of suspensions made up of either small inorganic particles or large organic molecules interpenetrated by a liquid.

Compounding Equipment for Topical Preparations

Equipment and materials needed for compounding topical dosage forms include the following:

- Electronic scales
- Compounding slabs
- Mortars and pestles
- Spatulas
- Alcohol

- Oil/water
- Powdered medications
- Creams
- Containers

Procedure for Compounding Topical Preparations

Ointments and creams are two semisolid external dosage forms that share common preparation techniques. Ointments are oil-based in nature, whereas creams are water-based. Seven steps must be followed to compound a topical dosage form:

1. Clean the glass slab.

2. Pour the desired amount of powder to compound into the ointment (Figure 10–17).

3. Add a partial amount of the cream needed to make the ointment (Figure 10–18).

4. Mix the powder into the cream so that they begin to form a single substance (Figure 10–19).

5. Continue to mix the powder and cream until the consistency is smooth, without any lumps or portions of dry powder remaining (Figure 10–20).

6. Put the blended ointment into the patient's ointment container (Figure 10–21).

7. Label the container with auxiliary labels such as "External Use Only" and "Refrigerate."

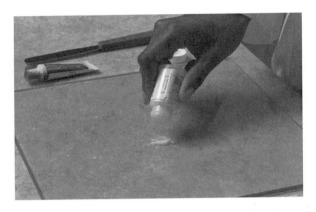

FIGURE 10–17   The technician pours the desired amount of powder into the ointment.

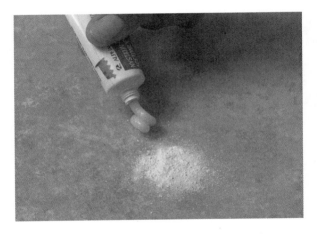

FIGURE 10–18   The technician adds a partial amount of the cream needed to make the ointment.

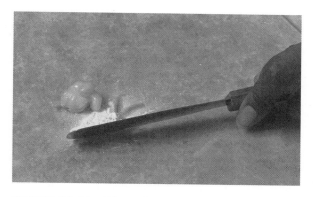

FIGURE 10–19   The technician mixes the powder into the cream.

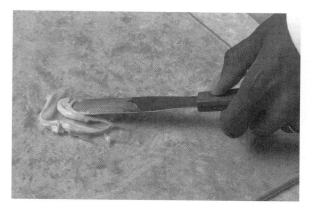

FIGURE 10–20   The technician blends the powder and cream.

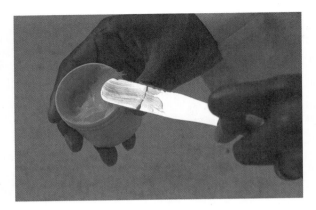

FIGURE 10–21   The technician puts the blended ointment into the patient's ointment container.

■ REPACKAGING

Because pharmaceutical manufacturers often prepare, package, and distribute commonly prescribed medications, the role of the pharmacy has changed from formulator, compounder, and packager to repackager of commercially available products. Drug packages must have four basic functions:

1. Protect their contents from deleterious environmental effects.

2. Protect their contents from deterioration resulting from handling.

3. Identify their contents completely and precisely.
4. Permit their contents to be used quickly, easily, and safely.

The package types most often found in hospital pharmacy departments include those used for:

- Oral solids
- Oral liquids
- Injections
- Respiratory medications
- Topical medications

Remember...

Compounded and repackaged products typically have short expiration dates, ranging from days to months. Expired compounded or repackaged medications cannot be returned, and must be disposed of.

UNIT-OF-USE PACKAGING

Unit-of-use packaging, sometimes referred to as "repackaging," is a suitable concept for inpatient or outpatient dispensing. An advantage to this type of dispensing process is that it allows the pharmacist to prepare medications for administration before their use is anticipated.

SINGLE-UNIT PACKAGING

Single-unit packages contain a single-dosage form. For example, only one tablet, or one capsule is contained in each single-unit package.

SINGLE-DOSE PACKAGING

A single-dose package is designed to hold a quantity of drug intended for administration as a single dose. Ampules are examples of single-dose injectable packaging.

AUTOMATED SYSTEMS

Fully automated systems are often used for repackaging oral solids, oral liquids, and injectables. The machines that are used to perform this work are controlled by a computer. The scope of this book is limited to machines used in pharmacy practice sites for work that includes:

- Storage
- Packaging
- Compounding
- Dispensing
- Distribution of medications
- Reduction of medication errors
- Improving documentation
- Enhancing security

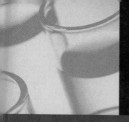

11

Sterile Compounding

Pharmaceutical compounding has been an integral part of pharmacy practice. Hospital pharmacy departments still perform some intravenous manufacturing, but the majority of parenteral products are prepared using commercially available medications and diluent solutions. ∎

ISSUES RELATED TO STERILE COMPOUNDING

For any institutional pharmacy setting that performs sterile compounding, the pharmacist must consider the following issues:

- Contamination: Maintain a clean area.
- Compatibility: Deal with problems of physical, chemical, and therapeutic incompatibilities.
- Stability: Establish a reasonable expiration date.
- Cost: Decrease drug costs.
- Errors: Reduce the potential for errors.
- Quality: Increase quality-control measures.
- Process: Ensure that orders and prescriptions are filled correctly.

Pharmaceutical compounding is increasing for the following reasons:

- The availability of dosage forms for most drugs is limited.
- The number of strengths of most drugs is limited, resulting from:
  - Drug shortages
  - Discontinued drugs
  - Orphan drugs
  - New therapeutic approaches
- Special patient populations (pediatrics, geriatrics, pain management) exist.
- Some drugs are unstable, and require preparation to be dispensed every few days.
- Patients may be allergic to excipients (inert substances used as diluents or drug vehicles) in commercially available products.

■ ROLE OF THE PHARMACY TECHNICIAN IN STERILE COMPOUNDING

The need for compounding pharmacists is increasing, and the responsibilities and opportunities for pharmacists and technicians are also increasing. Pharmacy technicians who engage in pharmaceutical compounding must expand their compounding knowledge and be trained at a higher skill level to perform the compounding responsibilities of sterile technique properly and safely.

Formal education of pharmacy technicians can take place either in institutional settings or academic programs. Sterile compounding is an advanced pharmacy technique that requires proper training of technicians, in addition to their general education. They must also receive proper orientation before being given this responsibility. During orientation, technicians should learn the following:

- Dressing correctly in approved garments
- Where and when to wash hands, and proper hand-washing techniques
- Personal hygiene techniques
- How to enter and leave controlled or critical areas
- The location of supplies and medications
- How to generate labels
- How to record orders
- How to document work, including which person handled dosing and what materials were used
- Types of drug information resources and their locations
- How to transmit medication orders
- How to store compounded sterile preparations
- How to send doses to patients
- How to reuse returned doses, if this is allowed
- Special procedures for TPN and chemotherapy
- Process validation, environmental monitoring, and other quality management
- Spill management and other problem resolution
- Safe staffing and scheduling

Remember...

The pharmacist maintains control over all pharmacy activities. Furthermore, the ultimate responsibility rests with the licensed pharmacist.

TYPES OF STERILE FORMULATIONS

Pharmacists or technicians will compound a wide variety of sterile formulations in different settings. These formulations will include products administered by injection, such as:

- Intravenous (IV)
- Intramuscular (IM)
- Subcutaneous (SC)
- Intradermal (ID)
- Intrathecal
- Epidural

There are also other sterile products, which may be administered by the following routes:

- Inhalation
- Intranasal
- Ophthalmic

EQUIPMENT FOR STERILE COMPOUNDING

The following equipment is essential for sterile compounding:

- Syringes and needles
- Alcohol pads
- Large-volume parenteral (LVP) solutions
- Small-volume parenteral (SVP) solutions
- Ampules or vials
- Laminar airflow hoods
- Refrigerators (with thermometers)
- Freezers
- Sinks with hot and cold water
- Automated compounding devices
- Disinfectant cleaning solutions
- Disposable, lint-free towels or wipes
- Disposable gowns, caps, masks, and sterile gloves
- Sharps containers
- Computer systems
- Shelving
- Carts
- Stainless steel furniture

- Adequate reference materials such as:
  - The latest edition of the *Handbook on Injectable Drugs*
  - Well-referenced compatibility and stability charts

■ LAMINAR AIRFLOW HOODS

Sterile products should be prepared in Class 100 environments, which can contain no more than 100 particles (a small piece or portion of anything, such as microorganisms) per cubic foot. These particles are 0.5 micron (or larger) in size. Laminar airflow hoods (LAHs) are commonly used to achieve a Class 100 environment. The required environmental control of aseptic areas has been made possible by the use of laminar airflow, originating through a high-efficiency particulate air (HEPA) filter. A laminar airflow hood is a cabinet-sized device that pushes room air through a HEPA filter. The HEPA filter pores are so fine that they filter out bacteria and produce sterilized air. Pharmacists or technicians use laminar airflow hoods to provide a bacteria-free environment for compounding intravenous solutions and other sterile prescription products (see Figures 11–1A and 11–1B).

The orientation for the direction of airflow can be horizontal or vertical. Great care must be exercised to prevent cross-contamination from one operation to another, especially with horizontal laminar airflow. Vertical laminar airflow hoods are used to prepare

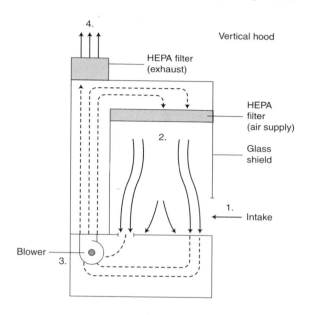

1. Room air enters the laminar airflow. This makes up about 30% of the air in the hood.

2. HEPA-filtered air enters and makes up 70% of the air in the hood.

3. Air from the work area is drawn down into the base and pulled back through the unit.

4. Air is exhausted after being filtered through carbon or HEPA filters.

FIGURE 11–1   (A) Vertical hood.

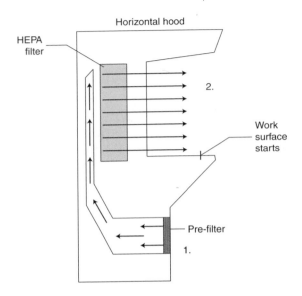

1. Room air enters, is filtered and drawn up to the top of the hood, where it is filtered through a HEPA filter.

2. Filtered air is directed out over the work surface.

FIGURE 11–1 **(B) Horizontal hood.**

drugs for chemotherapy. It is important for pharmacy technicians to keep their hands within the cleaned area of the hood as much as possible, and to not touch their hair, face, or clothing. Only materials essential for preparing the sterile product should be placed in the laminar airflow workbench or barrier isolator (see Figure 11–2).

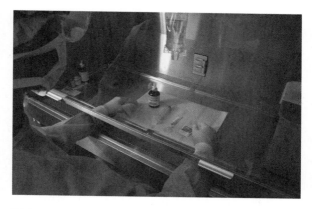

FIGURE 11–2   All materials being used in the laminar airflow hood must be placed within the workbench clean area.

Remember...

Checks of the air stream should be performed initially and at regular intervals (usually every six months) to be sure no leaks have developed through or around the HEPA filters.

Techniques for using laminar airflow hoods include:

- LAHs should be located away from all air currents that could introduce contaminants into them.
- LAHs should be turned on and allowed to run 15–30 minutes before they are used, so that they can blow out nonfiltered, nonsterile air that accumulated while the device was not in use.

- The HEPA filter should not come into contact with anything, including cleaning fluids, medications from syringes, and glass from medication containers such as ampules.

- Nothing should be put in the LAH except objects essential to the procedure.

- Jewelry should never be worn while working in the LAH.

- Talking, coughing, and unnecessary motions should not occur in the LAH, to avoid introducing contaminants.

- Smoking, eating, and drinking are prohibited.

- Aseptic activities should be performed at least six inches from the sides and front edge of the LAH.

- Airflow velocity and HEPA filter tests should be conducted at least every six months.

CLEANING LAMINAR AIRFLOW HOODS

Cleaning the laminar airflow hoods may be done with a non-shedding wipe or sponge dampened with Water for Injection, with or without mild detergent. This step should be followed by:

- Seventy percent isopropyl alcohol (or another appropriate disinfecting agent) should be used to clean all interior working surfaces before each use.

- A clean, lint-free cloth should be moved in a side-to-side motion, beginning at the rear and moving toward the front of the LAH.

- The walls of the LAH also must be cleaned from top to bottom with 70 percent isopropyl alcohol.

- This procedure should occur often throughout the compounding period and whenever the work surface becomes dirty.

- Because some materials require water to remove them, these materials may be first cleaned off with water, followed by the alcohol or other disinfecting agent.

- If the LAH has Plexiglas sides, they should be cleaned with warm, soapy water instead of alcohol.

- Spray bottles of alcohol or other disinfecting agents should never be used in the LAH.

- Once it is applied, alcohol should be allowed to air dry.

LARGE-VOLUME PARENTERAL SOLUTIONS

Large-volume parenteral (LVP) solutions are commonly stored in plastic or glass. Solutions for injection must be sterile, and contamination must be prevented by using aseptic techniques. LVP solutions are available in a variety of sizes (250 mL, 500 mL, 1000 mL).

Examples of LVP solutions with additives, manufactured in standard concentrations, include:

- Aminophylline
- Dopamine
- Lidocaine
- Nitroglycerin
- Potassium

In some cases, the preparation of LVPs by the pharmacist or technician depends on the drug and its intended use. The preparation of LVPs in the pharmacy must always follow aseptic technique.

Common examples of LVPs in use include:

- Dextrose Injection, USP
- Dextrose and Sodium Chloride Injection
- Amino Acid Injection
- Mannitol Injection, USP
- Ringer's Injection, USP
- Lactated Ringer's Injection, USP
- Sodium Chloride Injection, USP

These solutions are usually administered by intravenous infusion to replenish body fluids, electrolytes, or to provide nutrition. They are usually administered in volumes of 100 mL to 1 liter amounts (and more) per day by slow intravenous infusion with or without controlled-rate infusion systems.

When a patient is being maintained on parenteral fluids for several days, simple solutions providing adequate amounts of water, dextrose, and small amounts of sodium and potassium generally suffice. When patients are unable to take oral nutrition or fluids for several days or weeks, solutions of higher caloric content may be used (total parenteral nutrition). These admixtures are very useful for:

- Patients receiving chemotherapy
- Anorexic patients
- Pediatric patients

Remember...

Parenteral solutions must always be visually inspected after compounding and before use, and admixed solutions must be inspected after compounding.

SMALL-VOLUME PARENTERAL SOLUTIONS

Small-volume parenteral (SVP) solutions can be either directly administered to a patient or added to another parenteral formulation. Additive parenteral solutions are called "admixtures." SVP solutions can be supplied in different forms:

- Prefilled syringes
- Glass or plastic vials sealed with a rubber closure
- Ampules
- Plastic minibags or "piggybacks"

BASIC CONSIDERATIONS FOR STERILE COMPOUNDING

Pharmacy technicians must possess the following basic requirements to participate in sterile compounding:

- A working knowledge of the policy and procedure manuals for compounding, dispensing, and delivering sterile products
- Adequate training and adherence to hygienic and aseptic techniques
- Access to sufficient reference materials about sterile products

- Knowledge and awareness of the proper methods to store, label, and dispose of drugs and supplies

- Awareness of how to conduct sterile compounding in an area separate from other activities

- Knowledge of established procedures for assigning beyond-use dates that exceed the manufacturer-labeled expiration dates

USES FOR STERILE COMPOUNDING

In an institutional setting, the most common uses of sterile compounding include:

- Daily intravenous (IV) therapy
- Antibiotic piggybacks
- Total parenteral nutrition (TPN) solutions
- IV additives
- Preparation of pediatric dosage forms

ASEPTIC TECHNIQUE

Aseptic technique refers to the procedures used during preparation that maintain the sterility of pharmaceutical dosage forms. Sterilization is an essential concept in the preparation of sterile pharmaceutical products. Its aim is to provide a product that is safe and that eliminates the possibility of introducing infection.

Sterilization is a process used to destroy or eliminate viable microorganisms that may be present in or on a particular product or package. The process requires an overall understanding and control of all parts of the preparation for use of a particular product.

HAND WASHING

Hands must be washed properly, by using the correct technique. Proper hand washing depends on running water, a cleansing agent, and friction. The hands, fingernails, wrists, and forearms should be scrubbed under running water, with the fingertips pointing downward. Soap and friction are applied to the hands and wrists (see Figure 11–3).

Proper hand washing includes the following steps:

1. Remove all rings and wristwatches.

2. Stand close to, but not touching, the sink.

3. Turn on the faucet using a foot pedal or a dry, sterile towel. Discard the towel.

4. Wet hands, wrists, and forearms under running warm water, and apply liquid antibacterial soap.

5. For 15 to 30 seconds, scrub the palm of one hand with the fingers of the other hand, then repeat for the opposite hand.

6. Use a brush and scrub the fingernails and backs and palms of the hands, and then scrub the wrists and forearms.

7. Hold the hands in a downward position and rinse well.

8. Dry the hands and then the wrists gently with a sterile towel.

9. Use a dry, sterile towel to turn off the faucet if it is not operated by foot pedal.

CLEAN ROOM

A clean room is an area that is specially constructed and maintained to reduce the probability of environmental

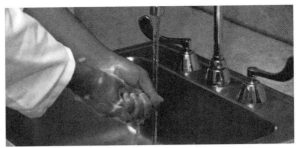

A

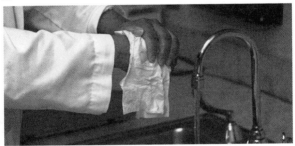

B

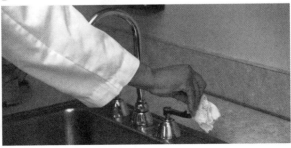

C

FIGURE 11–3   (A) The technician is washing her hands before the compounding procedure. (B) The hands must be dried. (C) If the faucet is not hands-free, use the towel to turn off the faucet to avoid recontaminating the hands.

contamination of sterile products during the manufacturing process. Clean rooms must meet the high standards of purity and cleanliness for parenteral compounding products, and must follow USP 797, which is a new and stringent set of rules and regulations regarding aseptic preparations.

USP 797 requires that the surfaces of all floors, walls, ceilings, cabinets, shelving, and work surfaces in the buffer room should be soft and smooth. These surfaces must also be free from crevices or cracks, making them easy to clean and sanitize.

Because air is one of the greatest potential sources of contaminants in clean rooms, special attention must be given to air being drawn into clean rooms by the following systems:

- Heating
- Ventilation
- Air conditioning

Personnel entering the aseptic area should enter only through an airlock. They should be attired in sterile coveralls with sterile hats, masks, goggles, and foot covers (see Figure 11–4). Traffic flow into the room should be minimized, and in-and-out movement rigidly restricted during a filling procedure. Clean rooms sometimes have an anteroom that is used for non-aseptic activities related to the clean room operation, such as:

- Gowning
- Handling of stock
- Order processing

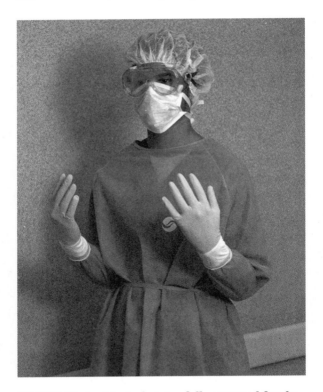

FIGURE 11–4   The technician fully prepared for the sterile procedure.

STERILE COMPOUNDING OF SOLUTIONS

A sterile product contains no living microorganisms. The need for sterility is based on the fact that through injection, the major body defense mechanisms are bypassed. In the hospital, a majority of patients will receive a medication that is administered by injection.

Examples of ophthalmic preparations that must be sterile include ointments, solutions, and suspensions. Sometimes pharmacy technicians must compound two solutions that are not commercially available. An example is the compounding of two materials that are both liquid in nature.

PROCEDURE FOR COMPOUNDING SOLUTIONS

The procedure for sterile compounding of solutions must be performed in the clean air space by using proper aseptic technique, as follows:

- Prepare all materials needed for the procedure.
- Swab the rubber tops of vials with alcohol and wait for them to dry.
- Pull the plunger back on the syringe slightly, then pull the amount needed to be drawn up.
- Insert the needle through the stopper.
- Push the air from the syringe into the vial.
- Withdraw the desired amount of medication.
- Withdraw the needle.
- Add the medication into the IV bag.
- Gently shake the bag of solution.
- Label the product of compounded solution.
- Store the product in the refrigerator.

COMPOUNDING AND DRUG-PREPARATION ERRORS

It is essential that pharmacy technicians take steps to decrease the risk of making an error when compounding and preparing medication products. These steps include:

- Read the product labels carefully.
- Do not process more than one prescription at a time.
- Label prescriptions properly.
- Store drugs properly.
- Maintain a safe work environment.
- Receive continuing education on changes in the pharmaceutical profession.

Remember...

Compounded medications often need preauthorization from insurance companies.

PACKAGING

There are several types of parenteral packaging:

- Syringes
- LVP solutions
- SVP solutions

■ LABELING

After a sterile product is prepared, it must be properly labeled to communicate the necessary information to ensure its appropriate use. Labels must:

- Be easily understood by a patient
- Avoid medical abbreviations or potentially confusing terminology
- Give clear directions for administering the product
- Be easily understood by other health-care professionals

■ STORAGE

Monitoring the storage conditions in the pharmacy is necessary to ensure that sterile products retain their respective quality attributes. Controlled-temperature storage areas such as refrigerators and freezers should be monitored at least once daily, with results documented on a temperature log.

■ QUALITY CONTROL AND QUALITY ASSURANCE

Quality control is the day-to-day assessment of all operations from the receipt of raw material to the distribution of the finished product.

Quality assurance is an oversight function, involving the adjusting of quality-control procedures and systems, with suggestions for changes as needed.

Each hospital should have written procedures covering the following:

- Handling and storage
- Preparing admixtures
- Labeling
- Transportation of IV fluids to the floors

Personnel involved in the preparation of IV admixtures should be trained and monitored on a regular basis. For quality control, documentation is essential and should include:

- Documentation of training procedures
- Quality-control results
- Laminar airflow hood certification
- Production records
- Concentration of all preparations

Quality-control documentation is required by various agencies and organizations.

12

Medication Errors

Medication use is a complex process that, at times, involves multiple organizations and professionals from various disciplines. A medication error is defined as any preventable event that causes or leads to inappropriate medication use or patient harm. Medication errors occur as a result of the actions of health-care professionals, patients, or consumers. ■

■ OCCURRENCE OF MEDICATION ERRORS

Medication errors may happen at anytime in any of the following places:

- Hospitals
- Physician offices
- Clinics
- Pharmacies
- Homes
- Operating rooms

Errors can also be made in the:

- Prescribing of medications
- Administering of medications
- Processes of diagnosing and testing

The Institute of Medicine estimates that at least 44,000 to as many as 98,000 Americans die each year as a result of medical errors, with 7,000 of these attributable to actual medication errors. Even when using the lower estimate of 44,000, deaths in hospitals due to medical errors exceed the deaths attributable each year to:

- Motor vehicle accidents (43,458)
- Breast cancer (42,297)
- AIDS (16,516)

Unquestionably, medication errors are one of the most common, avoidable causes of harm to patients. Medication errors may occur at three critical points:

- Prescribing
- Dispensing
- Administering

According to the National Institute of Medicine and other sources, most errors occur during the physician's ordering (39 percent) and the nurse's administration

(38 percent), with the remaining percentage of errors nearly equally divided between transcription and pharmacy dispensing.

Remember...

Medication errors can occur at the manufacturing level, as well as in hospitals, physicians' offices, or pharmacies.

■ PRESCRIBING ERRORS

Most medication errors occur in the ordering of prescriptions by physicians. Illegible handwriting by practitioners can cause the wrong drug to be given. Prescribing errors by physicians may be due to:

- Human factors (including mental alertness and memory lapses)
- Lack of drug knowledge
- Lack of patient information
- Rule violations (such as concealing a known medication error which has occurred)
- Inadequate monitoring
- Handwriting
- The use of some dangerous abbreviations

Remember...

Eliminating the usage of some dangerous abbreviations can play a significant role in reducing medication errors. These dangerous abbreviations include:

- U—Write out the word "units."
- QD—Write out the word "daily."
- QOD—Write out the phrase "every other day."
- QID—Write out the phrase "four times daily."

Also, use leading zeros before a decimal point, as follows: 0.2 mg, not ".2 mg".
Do not use trailing zeros, as follows: 2.0 mg should be written as "2 mg". (See Chapter 3.)

■ DISPENSING ERRORS

Medication errors can be made by pharmacists or pharmacy technicians. The following are factors that may cause medication errors in the pharmacy:

- Increased volume of work (The number of prescriptions doubled from 1992 to 2005.)
- Lack of patient counseling
- Lack of enough pharmacists
- Lack of adequate training for pharmacy technicians
- Human factors
- Difficulty in reading handwritten orders
- Confusion about different drugs with similar names, and differences between trade or brand and generic names

- Lack of information about a patient's drug allergies
- As a result of multiple, compounding events rather than from a single act by an individual
- Miscalculation of dosage or infusion rate
- Miscommunication (verbal or written)
- Mislabeling by manufacturer or pharmacist
- Environmental factors such as:
  - Noise
  - Poor lighting
  - Stress
  - Fatigue
- Poor management
- Computer error
- Growing problems with OTC drugs, herbal remedies, and purchasing medications via the Internet (which can often result in drug interactions due to improper cross-checking)

Remember...

Most experts agree that medication errors are due to a poor system, or some work-oriented or environmental condition, not from professional incompetence.

Remember...

Highly trained people make mistakes. Even if clinicians are well-educated and follow policies, procedures, or other guidelines, errors will still happen.

■ ADMINISTERING ERRORS

During administration of medication, errors may occur, whether nurses or other health-care personnel handle the administration. Factors that may cause administering errors, regardless of the person performing the administration, include:

- Human factors (including mental alertness and memory lapses)
- Lack of drug knowledge
- Lack of patient information
- Misuse of infusion pumps and other parenteral delivery systems
- Faulty drug identification or dose verification

Medication errors also may occur because of the following factors:

- Wrong drug
- Wrong dose
- Wrong patient
- Wrong time
- Wrong route
- Wrong technique
- Wrong information on the patient chart

Remember...

Dosing errors are the most common medication errors that occur in adults and children.

Remember...

The health-care provider who has the responsibility of administering a medication has the final opportunity to avoid a mistake.

THE PATIENT'S ROLE IN MEDICATION ERRORS

Medication errors may occur when patients self-administer drugs. Patients have a right to information regarding any proposed treatment, as well as the risks involved. The patient must be informed regarding his or her:

- Condition
- Treatment plan
- Prognosis
- Risks
- Benefits
- Alternative treatments

  As well as:

- Complications that may occur
- Other vital pieces of information

  Patients must have answers to the following questions explained to them to ensure safe medication use and to avoid medication errors:

- What are the brand and generic names of the medication?
- What is the purpose of the medication?

- What is the strength and dosage?
- What are the possible adverse effects, and what should be done if they occur?
- Are there medications that should be avoided while using this product?
- How long should this medication be used, and what outcomes are expected?
- When is the best time to take this medication?
- How should this medication be stored?
- What should be done if a dose is missed?
- What foods should be avoided while taking this medication?
- Does this medication replace another medication currently prescribed?
- What written information is available to explain this medication?

Patients can and should play an important role in their medication therapy. Education is critical, because patients can also make errors in administering medication.

Remember...

According to the Institute for Safe Medication Practices (ISMP), these are the most high-alert medications in which medication errors may occur:

- Insulin
- Narcotics and opiates
- Potassium chloride injections
- Heparin
- Concentrated sodium chloride (>0.9%)

■ AVOIDING MEDICATION ERRORS

Prevention of medication errors must be the most important priority of all health-care professionals, and those professionals must educate patients. Pharmacists and pharmacy technicians must do everything possible to prevent medication errors. The following items are essential for the technician to keep in mind:

- Confirm patient's identity
- Verify original prescription
- Verify medication calculation
- Communicate concerns
- Verify patient allergy history
- Inquire if patient has questions for pharmacist
- Maintain continuing education

Risk-reduction strategies for preventing errors include doing the following:

- Consult currently available drug reference texts.
- Document essential patient information, including:
  - Allergies
  - Age
  - Weight
  - Current diagnoses
  - Current medication regimen
- Require clarification of any order that is incomplete or illegible.

Human factors that increase the risk of medication errors and are preventable include:

- Fatigue
- Alcohol and/or the use of other drugs
- Illness
- Distractions
- Emotional states
- Unfamiliar situations or problems

Other factors include:

- Equipment design flaws
- Inadequate labeling or instructions
- Communication problems
- Hard-to-read handwriting
- Unsafe work conditions

■ MEDICATION ERROR REPORTING

Reporting medication errors and problems with products should be mandatory. However, reporting medication errors is totally voluntary. There are two medication error reporting systems:

- FDA MedWatch Programs
- United States Pharmacopoeia's (USP) Medication Error Reporting Program

FDA MEDWATCH PROGRAM

The FDA's MedWatch program encourages the voluntary reporting of adverse events or product problems.

MedWatch allows health-care professionals and consumers to report serious suspected problems via the following:

- By telephone: (800) FDA-1088
- By fax: (800) FDA-0178
- Through the Internet at: http://www.fda.gov

MedWatch also provides important and timely clinical information about safety issues involving products, including:

- Prescription and OTC drugs
- Biologics
- Medical and radiation-emitting devices
- Special nutritional products, such as:
  - Medical foods
  - Dietary supplements
  - Infant formulas

Pharmacists and technicians can join an electronic mailing list to get up-to-date information that the FDA disseminates. They can also receive information as a result of information reported to MedWatch at the e-mail address noted earlier.

USP'S MEDICATION ERROR REPORTING PROGRAM

This program is presented in cooperation with the Institute for Safe Medication Practices (ISMP), and provides practitioners the opportunity to share medication error experiences through a nationwide network to help understand why errors occur, and how to prevent them. Educational information gained from the program helps health-care professionals avoid errors by recognizing circumstances and causes of actual and potential errors.

Remember...

Reporting is confidential and can be anonymous. Reports may be phoned to (800) 23-ERROR [800-233-7767] or faxed to (301) 816-8532. More information can be found at http://www.usp.org

MINIMIZING LIABILITY

Upon detecting an error in dispensing, the pharmacy technician must take all necessary steps to rectify it promptly and notify the pharmacist immediately. Failure to do so can subject the pharmacist to punitive damage liability in addition to actual damage for the injury caused. Immediately upon discovery, the pharmacist should inform the patient and the prescribing physician of the prescription error.

◼ NEGLIGENCE AND MALPRACTICE PENALTIES

Pharmacy laws are designed to protect the public by ensuring that a knowledgeable individual double-checks the results of the prescribing process and oversees the use of medications. Pharmacy technicians should be familiar with the workplace's policies and procedures manual. Technicians must also receive training on the job. The Joint Commission requires organizations to prove that their personnel are competent.

Technicians and pharmacists need to be informed about prevention of medication errors. In addition to the institution's or the company's liability, pharmacists and technicians may be held accountable for their negligence, malpractice, and penalties due to a medication error that involves the injury to, or death of, a patient.

The failure to do something that a reasonable person might do, or doing something that a reasonable person might not do, is termed "negligence." A pharmacist or a supervised pharmacy technician who violates a regulation or law that establishes a standard of care, and a standard that is designed to protect patients, may be guilty of negligence.

Negligence of a professional, such as a pharmacist, or a pharmacist-supervised technician, is termed "malpractice." A pharmacist who fails to perform a prospective drug regimen review, gives incorrect advice, or doesn't warn a patient about potential adverse effects is guilty of malpractice.

Penalties concerning negligence or malpractice may include:

- Restrictions on practice
- Suspension of ability to practice
- Fines
- Revocation of ability to practice
- Jail sentences

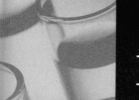

13

Computer Systems in the Pharmacy

Computers constitute a major technology that supports the practice of pharmacy. Computers are data processors. They receive input, and then process and produce output.

Pharmacists and technicians are assisted by computers to deliver the following:

- Correct information
- Correct patient
- Correct time
- Correct place
- Correct format
- Correct medication ▪

■ COMPONENTS OF A COMPUTER SYSTEM

Computers can be readily understood by looking at the following five components of a computer system:

1. Computer inputs:
   - Keyboard
   - Mouse (trackball)

- Microphones (to record sounds, or for use in speech-recognition software)
- Public kiosks (touch screens)

2. Computer outputs:
   - Monitor or display
   - Speakers
   - Printers
   - Plotters

3. Memory (random access memory, or RAM)

4. Storage includes the following devices:
   - Hard drives
   - Floppy drives
   - Removable data cartridges
   - Read-write CD-ROM drives

5. Processor of the computer (the brain of the workstation)

■ COMPUTER SYSTEM DATABASES

At the core of nearly every pharmacy software program is a **database application**. In pharmacy management, multiple databases usually are being managed. Database applications can include:

- Patient and customer profiles
- Prescriber profiles
- Drugs, including drug interactions and other essential drug information
- Pricing

- Billing
- Payers
- Inventory management

PATIENT AND CUSTOMER PROFILES

Computer system databases allow the pharmacist and technician to have complete information about their customers and patients, including:

- Prescribers
- Medication history
- Medical history (drug allergies and drug interactions)
- Insurers

PRESCRIBER PROFILES

The computer can provide information about the prescribers, including:

- State identification numbers
- Affiliation with facilities
- Insurers

DRUG DATABASES

Drug databases help pharmacy personnel access the following information:

- Brand names
- Generic equivalents
- Adverse effects
- Dosing
- Dosage forms

- Kinetics
- Pregnancy risks
- Potential interactions

Remember...

Competency with electronic drug databases is an expectation within the pharmacy profession today.

PRICING DATABASES

Most pricing databases offer pharmacy personnel the following benefits:

- Drug-pricing analysis
- Formulary management using drug subsets, sub-classes, etc.
- Easy-to-use format
- Accurate pricing based on the National Drug Data File (NDDF)
- Powerful drug-classification systems
- Time-saving drug data updating and maintenance

BILLING DATABASES

The database can electronically manage third-party information, including:

- HMOs and insurers
- The authorization of third-party transactions
- Credit cards

PAYER DATABASES

Payer databases offer a wide array of information, including:

- Payments
  - Amounts
  - Arrangements
  - Delays
  - Forms of payment
  - Schedule forms
  - Share of costs
- Payer of last resort
  - Medicaid as secondary payer
  - Authorization requests

INVENTORY MANAGEMENT

Computers can manage inventory information by:

- Adjusting inventory as prescriptions are filled
- Automatically reordering based on inventory levels
- Analyzing turnover
- Generating purchase orders
- Tracking costs
- Identifying inventory to be discarded, or outdated inventory
- Noting items borrowed from other pharmacies

Pharmacy technicians play an active role in inventory and narcotic control. Most computer systems provide separate controls for Schedule II drugs. Appropriate security clearance is important for narcotic-control records, and access should be limited to the pharmacists and technicians involved with record keeping.

■ COMPUTER SYSTEM FUNCTIONS

Pharmacy computer systems help pharmacy staff members to greatly reduce the use of paper, and to process prescriptions more safely. This helps save time and money, and increases pharmacy profits by streamlining operations.

MANAGEMENT FUNCTIONS

The computer system is able to process data that serve to improve efficiencies in running the pharmacy day-to-day business affairs. Some of the functions provided by the computer system related to pharmacy management are the following:

- Report distribution of narcotic use records
- Create financial reports (billing information)
- Maintain files
- Reduce data workloads

LABELING

Computers are also able to provide:

- Labels
- Receipts
- Customer information for instructions about the use of medication

BAR CODES

Bar codes are a unique arrangement of lines that are used to identify particular items in drug products:

- Drug name
- Drug strength
- Dosage form
- Lot number
- Expiration date

Bar codes help technicians ensure that a patient receives the:

- Correct drug
- Correct dose

Remember...

Bar codes present information in a manner that a computer can read. Technicians should not rely solely on bar codes. They must check their work to ensure accuracy and appropriateness.

TECHNOLOGY AND HIPAA

The Health Insurance Portability and Accountability Act (HIPAA) of 1996 mandates:

- Privacy for health information
- Standards for electronic transactions of health information
- Security of electronic health information
- National identifiers for the patient in health-care transactions

HIPAA regulations also provide patients with better access to their own medical records. Patients always have the right to:

- Request access to information
- Request amendments of protected health information
- Request alternative communications
- Request accounting of disclosures
- Request additional restriction of information

Remember...

Other technologies, such as prescriber order entry, actually complement HIPAA regulations and provide additional incentives for moving toward electronic medical record implementation.

DOCUMENTATION

The documentation component of health care has been one of the reasons pharmacy has struggled with obtaining provider status in Medicare regulations and other private sector circumstances. By using a computer system, you are able to review all documentation that you have already provided. Therefore, computer systems help offer:

- Unique patient identification
- Accuracy
- Completeness
- Timeliness
- Interoperability across documentation systems

- The ability to conduct audits
- Confidentiality
- Security

AUTOMATION

Automation, in general, means that machines are used to perform work. These machines are usually controlled by a computer. The scope of this book is limited to machines used in pharmacy practice sites for work that includes:

- Storage
- Counting
- Packaging
- Improved inventory management
- Compounding
- Dispensing
- Cost savings
- Labeling dosage forms
- Distribution of medications
- Improved accuracy based on bar code recognition
- Improved efficiency of dispensing functions
- Ability to track expiration dates
- Reduction of medication errors
- Collecting, controlling, and maintaining transaction information

Remember...

Pharmacy technicians play an important role in managing a variety of computerized systems and automation technologies. This enables the pharmacist to have more time for direct patient-care activities.

14

Pharmacy Operation

The first role of management for any business enterprise should be to establish the objectives and goals for the organization. Pharmacy managers must provide the policies and procedures that serve as the framework for accomplishing the stated objectives. For pharmacy operation, the manager must provide a sense of direction by setting guidelines for current and future activities. ▪

■ THE ROLE OF THE PHARMACY MANAGER

Pharmacy practice has changed dramatically over the last several years. Therefore, the need for pharmacy managers has increased. Managers are responsible for:

- Planning
- Organizing
- Controlling resources
- Productivity
- Quality
- Service
- Price

Remember...

The pharmacy manager is responsible for and accountable for the finances of the pharmacy.

PROFITABILITY OF THE PHARMACY PRACTICE

Without establishing the pharmacy's business practices so that it makes a regular profit, pharmacy managers cannot achieve the pharmacy's ultimate goal of serving the community. The pharmacy technician must follow the business and financial goals and objectives of the pharmacy, and help ensure that receipts are greater than expenses. The technician is engaged in some parts of pharmacy operation, and must understand the importance of the following concepts:

- Cost
- Overhead
- Markup
- Discount
- Inventory control

COST

The overall cost for the pharmacy may include the cost of:

- Drug purchases
- Salaries
- Operating expenses
- Utilities

- Business insurance and liability
- Net profit

Remember...

The net profit for each drug sold is calculated as the difference between the overall cost and the selling price.

The effects of costs in the institutional pharmacy or community pharmacy depend on the following factors:

- Output or volume
- Quality of services
- Scope of services
- Relative efficiency

An increase in cost will occur as a result of an increase in one of the preceding factors. It is important to understand the effect of a change in one or more of these factors.

OVERHEAD

Pharmacy overhead may include any of the following:

- Accounting, legal, and professional fees
- Cleaning, repairs, and security
- Computer systems, maintenance, and software
- Corporate overhead (such as central management)
- Depreciation
- Federal and state regulation compliance fees (for example, HIPAA)

- Insurance, taxes, and licenses
- Interest paid on pharmacy-related debt
- Marketing and advertising
- Rent or mortgage
- Utilities (air conditioning, heat, lighting, water, telephones)

MARKUP

The term **markup** refers to the difference between the cost of merchandise and its selling price. Markup is sometimes called "margin of profit" or "gross profit." The markup is the amount of the retailer's sale price minus the purchase price. For example, if a medication costs $8.00 per package, and the markup is 50%, the pharmacy's price to consumers will be: $8.00 + $4.00 markup (which is $8.00 × 50%), for a total of $12.00.

Remember...

For calculating the markup rate, you may use this formula:

$$\text{Markup rate} = \frac{\text{Markup}}{\text{Cost}} \times 100\%$$

DISCOUNT

The purpose of discounting is to present all costs in their present value, and to incorporate society's time preference for money. We all have a preference for when we would like to receive money. Most of us would rather receive $10 today rather than $10 a year from now.

Pharmacies may give a 5% to 10% discount on the price of a prescription to a special group of patients (that is, senior citizens). Sometimes the discount is limited to prescriptions purchased on certain days of the week.

Example:

An elderly patient is paying for a prescription for Zocor 20 mg for one month (#30). The usual price for 30 tablets is $158.99. If this patient qualifies for a 10% discount, how much will the patient pay?

10% of 158.99 = 158.99 × 1/10 = $15.899, which rounds up to $15.90

Now subtract: 158.99 − 15.90 = $143.09

The patient will pay a discounted price of $143.09.

INVENTORY CONTROL

Inventory may be defined as a list of merchandise, itemized by various types, and its costs. The goal of sound inventory management in today's environment is a reasonable turnover of products combined with:

- Rapid billing
- Receiving
- Minimal waste

The duties and responsibilities of pharmacy technicians regarding inventory control include the following:

- Maintaining an adequate stock of medication
- Accounting
- Keeping adequate medical equipment

- Ordering supplies
- Order verification

INVENTORY SYSTEMS

A pharmaceutical inventory system is able to:

- Control inventory
- Forecast needs
- Initiate reorders

> **Remember...**
>
> The goal of a good inventory system is to ensure that the correct amount of stock is available at all times.

The inventory system may be computerized. Computerized inventory systems automatically are able to adjust inventory and generate orders based on maintaining set inventory levels.

PERPETUAL INVENTORY

Perpetual inventory systems allow review of drug use on a monthly basis. They allow pharmacists to conduct monthly drug use reviews, and monitor the budget. Board regulations require perpetual inventories of each Schedule II controlled substance that has been received, dispensed, or disposed of. These perpetual inventories must be reconciled every 10 days in some states.

POINT OF SALE

The point of sale (POS) is an inventory control system that allows inventory to be tracked as it is used. It is the most suitable, flexible, and open-ended system on the market. The POS master can increase overall profitability. These systems can handle:

- Significant volumes of customers and transactions
- Orders
- Credits
- Inter-store transfers
- Returns

INVENTORY TURNOVER RATES

Turnover is the rate at which inventory is used or the number of days it takes for the complete stock of an item to be used. For higher-cost pharmaceuticals, this value may be used to prevent excessive expenditures by the pharmacy. For example, certain vaccines or drugs have short expiration dates, so you would not want to stock a lot of them since they would expire quickly. *Inventory turnover rate* is a mathematical calculation of the number of times the average inventory is replaced over a period of time, usually annually.

Inventory turnover is calculated using the following formula:

Cost of Goods Sold from Stock Sales (during the past 12 months) ÷ Average Inventory Investment (during the past 12 months)

Annual Cost of Goods Sold	Inventory Investment	Annual Inventory Turns
$10,000	$10,000	1
$10,000	$5,000	2
$10,000	$2,500	4

Remember...

Inventory turnover is based on the cost of items (what you paid for them), not sales dollars (what you sold them for).

To understand the concept of inventory turnover, consider the following:

- You sell $10,000 worth of a product (your cost) each year.
- Total revenue received from sales of this product is $12,500.
- If you bought the entire $10,000 worth of the product on January 1st, at the end of the year you would have made a $2,500 gross profit on your $10,000 investment.

- Other choices include buying $5,000 worth of the product on January 1st and buying an add additional $5,000 worth of the product in the middle of the year.

- Or, you could choose to buy $2,500 worth of the product two more times during the year after your initial purchase of $5,000 worth of the product.

- Your gross profit would be the same at the end of the year, but with this alternate method of purchasing, you have freed up $7,500 to be used for other purposes during the year.

AUTOMATED WORK SYSTEMS

Automated work systems are desirable because they are capable of achieving far superior efficiency and accuracy compared to any other system, in appropriate applications. Their primary use is for the functions of:

- Counting
- Packaging
- Labeling dosage forms

Remember...

Pharmacy technicians must have proper training, and be familiar with a computer to operate automated work systems.

■ ORDERING

One of the simplest and most widely used methods of inventory control is a **want book**. A want book is simply a list of items that the pharmacy or technician needs to order. Information to be specified when ordering includes the following:

- Item name and manufacturer. (For a drug product, the generic or brand name must be specified.)
- Strength and dosage form of the drug. (If ordering a device, the size must be included.)
- Quantity of drug dosage forms per package (such as, bottle of 100, package of 3).
- Type of packaging.
- Number of bottles, devices, or packages being ordered.

   Remember...

   Proper record keeping is essential for inventory control, recall tracking, and patient safety.

■ PURCHASING PROCEDURES

Purchasing procedures must be started after understanding the factors related to cost. In the hospital, usually there are two types of purchasing systems, as follows:

- Independent purchasing
- Group purchasing

Remember...

Generally, the director of pharmacy or the pharmacy buyer handles purchasing. Pharmacy technicians are sometimes involved in purchasing in the community (retail) pharmacy.

PRICING

Pharmacy technicians are sometimes involved in the process of pricing. There are three basic pricing mechanisms:

- Percentage markup system
- Dispensing fee
- Markup fee system

AVERAGE WHOLESALE PRICE

Average wholesale price (AWP) is the average of the prices charged by the national drug wholesalers for a given product. Pharmacy computers can be programmed to automatically calculate the usual and customary price when a prescription is filled. Therefore, the selling price of a drug is calculated by using the following formula:

Selling price of drug = AWP + Professional fee

The following chart determines the professional fee:

AWP	Professional Fee
Less than $20.00	$4.00
$20.01 to $50.00	$5.00
$50.01 and higher	$6.00

Example:

If the AWP for 30 capsules of Cefanex 500 mg is $5.65, the corresponding professional fee (because $5.65 is less than $20.00) would be $4.00. To calculate the retail price, use this formula:

$5.65 + $4.00 = $9.65

REPACKAGING

The role of the pharmacist and the pharmacy technician has changed from formulator and packager to repackager of commercially prepared medications. Pharmacists and pharmacy technicians repackage bulk containers of medication into patient-specific containers of medication—this is called "unit-of-use packaging." The unit-dose system of dispensing medication in organized healthcare settings has been the driving force behind repackaging programs.

Technicians may manually repackage a medication or use a unit-dose packaging machine. Medications that are commonly repackaged include:

- Tablets
- Capsules
- Liquids
- Powders
- Ointments
- Respiratory products

Remember...

Proper procedures for repackaging (regardless of the dosage form) must be followed to ensure that the final package has the same product in a properly labeled, appropriate package.

Drug packages must have four basic functions:

- Protect contents from deleterious environmental effects.
- Protect contents from deterioration resulting from handling.
- Identify contents completely and precisely.
- Permit contents to be quickly, easily, and safely used.

■ DISPOSAL OF DRUGS

Disposal requirements for expired drugs are listed in the package inserts or on a material safety data sheet (MSDS). Expired, deteriorated, contaminated, or other nonreusable drug products should be removed immediately from usable pharmacy stock and disposed of.

Expired drugs should be placed into containers labeled with "Expired Drugs—DO NOT USE," "RETURNED FOR CREDIT—DO NOT USE," or a similar warning that can be clearly understood. Expired drugs and their disposal methods must always be documented. Drugs that should be disposed of include:

- Parenteral medications
- Oral liquids and solids
- Ophthalmic solutions and suspensions
- Nasal solutions
- Ointments
- Creams
- Topical solutions
- Biologicals
- Suppositories
- Transdermal patches
- Insulin
- Inhalers
- Tablets
- Capsules

ACCOUNTING

Accounting is a system of monitoring the financial status of a facility and the financial results of its activities. Accounting may be divided into two major categories:

- Financial
- Managerial

Pharmacies utilize a variety of ways to monitor financial accounts and the total financial operations of the business. The majority of pharmacies rely on accounting software packages to prepare financial records. A computerized accounting system is the most common method used in pharmacies today.

BILLING

Some pharmacies do their own in-house billing. Therefore, pharmacy technicians must be familiar with how to bill patients or insurers, and must follow the policies and procedures of the pharmacy.

INVOICES

An **invoice** is a paper describing a purchase and the amount due. Invoices should be placed in a special folder until paid. Most invoices are due within 30 days after receipt of product. Some vendors will send a statement that details all purchases that have been sent within a certain period, while others invoice each shipment separately and expect payment within the 30-day period after a shipment is delivered.

RECEIVING

Receiving is one of the most important parts of the pharmacy operation. When products that have been ordered arrive at the pharmacy, it is essential that a system for checking purchases and receiving them be in place. Generally, the individual who ordered the products should not handle receiving those products. All items must be carefully checked against the purchase order. The following procedures should be followed:

- Verification and comparison against the purchase order for:
  - Name of product
  - Quantity of boxes
  - Package size
  - Any gross damage to boxes or containers
- For drug products, the following must be checked:
  - Generic name and brand name
  - Dosage form
  - Size of the package
  - Strength
  - Quantity
  - Expiration date

■ BAR CODING

Bar coding is becoming increasingly popular in the pharmacy setting, although its use has been delayed because of the lack of a universal bar code standard for all medication. Bar coding all pharmaceuticals in a uniform, consistent manner will help to offer the following:

- Product-specific, manufacturer-generated bar codes
- Product-specific, pharmacy-system-generated bar codes
- Pharmacy information-system-generated bar codes

Remember...

Bar coding saves dollars, time, and, most important, lives by helping reduce medication errors.

RETURNING PRODUCTS

The manufacturer or wholesaler should be notified immediately of damaged or incorrect shipments or expired medications. A return merchandise authorization also should be requested to return the rejected shipment.

DRUG RECALLS

Drug recall is a process of retrieving defective drugs once they have been shipped from the manufacturer. Reasons for drug recalls include:

- Mislabeling
- Packing the wrong drug
- Packing the wrong dose in a bottle
- Adulteration of the drug product

The pharmacy manager must establish a written procedure detailing how to handle recalled products. The policy and procedures manual should address such items as:

- Identifying the recalled product
- Locating the product in the pharmacy
- Quarantining and returning the product

RECORD KEEPING

Several reasons for maintaining the records in the pharmacy are becoming increasingly important, including:

- Legal
- Financial
- Professional

Record keeping is required by law regarding the acquisition and disposition of drugs. Record keeping is also required for patient utilization of drugs, or for the past and present financial status of the pharmacy.

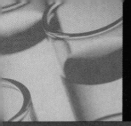

15

Billing and Health Insurance

Developing accurate and efficient documentation and billing systems are clinical, legal, and economic mandates for the pharmacy profession. Billing involves detailing the services that have been provided, along with any laboratory tests performed in the pharmacy. Today, most prescriptions are paid for by third-party payers. ■

PAYMENT

Pharmacy technicians must bill the patient without error to guarantee timely payment. Proper coding for treatment is vital to the financial management of a pharmacy. The processing of payment requests must include:

- Patient's legal name
- Relationship to insured (self, spouse, child, other)
- Address and telephone number
- Individual identification number
- Employer of insured party
- Claims address, department, proper P.O. box
- Date of service

- Diagnostic codes (that support treatment)
- Treatment codes
- Date of birth

There are several methods of payment for prescriptions, as follows:

1. Direct payment by the patient
2. Reimbursement from a governmental program
3. Reimbursement from a nongovernmental program

The pharmacy technician must be familiar with the following terms and their definitions regarding health insurance:

- **Birthday rule:** This determines the primary payer when the patient is a child living with both parents and each parent carries health insurance. The parent with the earlier birthday in the calendar year (month and day) is the primary insurer for the dependent children.
- **Clean claim:** Error-free insurance claim.
- **Co-pay, co-payment:** Amount of money the patient owes at each visit; this varies with insurers from $5 to $25 or more.
- **Coinsurance:** The amount or percentage the insured is responsible for after the deductible has been met.
- **Deductible:** Amount of money paid out-of-pocket by the patient at the beginning of each calendar year before health insurance benefits begin to cover claims.

- **Explanation of benefits (EOB):** Document sent from the insurance company to the patient outlining payments made to physicians, write-offs, and any patient responsibilities.

- **Health Maintenance Organization (HMO):** Organization that provides services to covered persons in an individual, group, or public health plan.

- **Insurance premium:** The amount of money, often paid monthly by a policyholder or insured, to an insurance company to obtain coverage.

- **Third-party payer:** An individual or organization that is not directly involved in an encounter, but has a connection because of its obligation to pay, in full or in part, for that encounter. Three third-parties are the following:

  Party #1: The health-care provider

  Party #2: The patient

  Party #3: The insurance carrier

- **Preferred Provider Organization (PPO):** A type of health insurance coverage in which physicians provide health-care services to members of the plan at a discount.

- **Preauthorization:** The insurance company reviews the treatment plan and will agree to authorize and pay for treatment.

- **Preferred provider:** Physicians and pharmacists who contract with insurance carriers to provide patient care at a discounted rate.

CODING SYSTEM

The purpose of coding is to make every effort to ensure clear and concise communication among all parties involved. In most cases, these parties are health-care providers and the insurance companies (third-party payers).

Pharmacy technicians need to be familiar with the following terms and forms:

- **CPT codes:** Common Procedural Terminology codes are used to describe clinical interactions with patients and their services and procedures. These codes can be varied because of the following reasons:

  - The patient is new.
  - The clinical situation is complex.
  - The amount of time the pharmacist or technician must spend with each patient differs.

- **ICD-9-CM codes:** The International Classification of Diseases, Ninth Revision, Clinical Modification, is a set of standard numbers used for designating patients' diseases. The physician makes the diagnosis of the patient's conditions, and the pharmacist must simply obtain the correct ICD-9 code from the physician to use on the reimbursement forms.

- **HCPCS codes:** Health Care Finance Administration Common Procedure Coding System (HCPCS) codes may be used for billing medical devices such as medication-administration sets, syringes, walkers, and wheelchairs. The majority of entries described in the HCPCS code book apply to supplies and medications. These codes are used by most

Medicare/Medicaid carriers for reporting these items, rather than the codes listed under "special supplies" in the medicine section of CPT-4.

Remember...

The HCPCS codes often identify the name of the supply or drug, its dosage, and its strength.

UNDERSTANDING INSURANCE POLICIES

Pharmacy technicians must understand the insurance companies' rules and policy guidelines. In reviewing various insurance carriers, you need to recognize the various ways a patient may obtain insurance coverage, as follows:

- **Group health plan:** A plan arranged by an employer or special interest group for the benefit of members and their eligible dependents.

- **Individual or personal plan:** A plan issued to an individual. This type of coverage has a high premium.

- **Prepaid health-care program:** A plan whereby services are rendered by physicians or facilities who elect to participate in a set program for services.

INSURANCE HEALTH PLANS

Most patients are in some type of health-care plan, so pharmacists now have multiple participation agreements and plans when providing services to patients.

BLUE CROSS AND BLUE SHIELD

Several insurance carriers conduct business within the United States. One of the largest of these is the Blue Cross/Blue Shield group. Although many people consider Blue Cross/Blue Shield to be separate or different from many other companies, in truth, their contracts cover many of the same procedures and have many of the same benefits as other indemnity plans.

Blue Cross is an insurance plan that covers:

- Inpatient hospital services
- Nursing home services
- Home health-care services

Blue Shield is the portion of a patient's insurance that provides financial assistance with outpatient costs for services such as physician charges.

TRICARE

TRICARE is the U.S. Department of Defense Military Health System (formerly called the Civilian Health and Medical Program of the Uniformed Services, or CHAMPUS). It is a federal program to assist active duty military personnel and eligible dependents as well as retirees and their eligible dependents with the cost of medical expenses.

CHAMPVA

CHAMPVA is the Civilian Health and Medical Program of the Veterans Administration that provides a medical benefit program for spouses and children of veterans with total, permanent, service-connected disabilities, or for the surviving dependents of veterans who die as a result of service-connected disabilities.

Remember...

Members who receive TRICARE benefits do not qualify for coverage under CHAMPVA.

Remember...

Claims must be submitted to CHAMPVA's main office in Denver, Colorado, either electronically, or on the CMS-1500 form for services.

MEDICARE

Medicare is a national health insurance program for:

- Persons over the age of 65
- Qualified disabled persons
- Blind persons

There are four parts to the Medicare program. Because each program has different policies regarding payment and coverage, separate organizations are responsible for processing claims. These programs include:

- **Medicare Part A:** provides coverage for inpatient care, such as:
  - Hospitals
  - Nursing homes
  - Skilled nursing facilities
  - Hospices
  - Some home health services
- **Medicare Part B:** programs under the direction of private insurance carriers that have placed bids with the government to become intermediaries. Part B covers physicians and non-physician professionals

as listed in the following, as well as the included types of services:

- Physicians in both inpatient and outpatient settings
- Nurses
- Nurse midwives
- Prescribing advanced practice nurses
- Physician assistants
- Therapists, such as speech therapists
- Podiatrists
- Clinical psychologists
- Diagnostic testing
- Durable equipment management (DEM)
- Supplies
- Home health services

Remember...

Part A does not require a monthly premium for coverage. Medicare Part B recipients must pay a monthly premium for continued coverage.

Remember...

Some Medicare Advantage Plans may pay all or part of the Medicare Part B premium. A plan that offers this benefit may save the patient money. All Medicare Part A and Part B services are covered.

- **Medicare Part C:** This is the Medicare advantage portion, and includes coverage in one of the following:
  - HMO
  - PPO
  - Similar organizations

Remember...

> If a Medicare beneficiary selects the coverage of Part C, they are required to receive services according to the selected carrier's arrangements.

- **Medicare Part D:** In an effort to provide better health coverage for Medicare beneficiaries, starting in 2006, Medicare beneficiaries began receiving limited coverage for prescription drug benefits. Medicare Part D is also called the **Medicare Prescription Drug Plan**. This plan is available to all people with Medicare to help lower prescription drug costs and help protect against higher costs in the future. Medicare prescription drug coverage is insurance wherein private companies provide the coverage.

Remember...

> Medicare will help employers and unions continue to provide retiree drug coverage that meets Medicare's standards.

Medicare Health Insurance Card (HIC)

A Medicare health insurance card is issued to every person who is entitled to Medicare benefits and may be identified by its red, white, and blue coloring. This card indicates which type of coverage the patient has, as follows:

- Part A (hospital)
- Part B (medical, physician services)
- Part C (HMO, PPO)
- Part D (prescription drugs)

The card identifies the Medicare beneficiary and includes the following information:

- Name as it appears on the Social Security records
- Medicare Health Insurance Claim Number (HICN)
- Beginning date of Medicare entitlement for particular services
- Gender
- Place for beneficiary signature

Medicare Modernization Act of 2003 (MMA)

This act was the largest expansion of Medicare since 1965. Its long-awaited changes focus on improving health care for senior citizens by providing them with prescription drug benefits and more health-care choices. The plan provides the following:

- Drug discount cards that offer up to 25% savings per prescription.
- Low-income senior citizens may receive up to $600 to help pay for drugs.

- Reorganization of the rules of out-of-pocket expenses.
- Catastrophic coverage after $3,600 of expenses are incurred.
- No premiums or deductibles from those seniors with incomes of less than 150% of the federal poverty line.
- Reduced costs for both generic and brand name drugs.
- Employers receive varying government subsidies for the drug costs of their retirees.
- Establishment of HSAs (Health Savings Accounts) that may be funded in a variety of ways.
- Increases Medicare payments to rural providers and hospitals.
- Improvements in the Medicare claims appeals process.

MEDICAID

Medicaid is a state-funded assistance program created to help alleviate some of the expenses of medical care for qualified recipients.

Remember...

Medicaid is not an insurance program.

Medicaid is available to the following recipients:
- Certain low-income families
- Some elderly patients (65 years of age or older)

- Blind persons
- Disabled persons
- Dependent children who have been deprived of the support of at least one parent
- Those who are financially eligible

■ INSURANCE FORMS

An insurance coverage form is used by many practices to verify insurance coverage and document this information. There are three types:

- The superbill (also known as a charge slip)
- The CMS-1500
- The patient claim form

Remember...

The Centers for Medicare and Medicaid Services form (CMS-1500) is a standardized form approved by both the American Medical Association and CMS for use as a "universal" form for billing professional services.

CMS-1500 FORMS

When deciding whether to use the CMS-1500 form to bill for pharmacist care services, the pharmacist or technician should consider the nature of the services, as well as the payer to whom the claim will be submitted. Pharmacists use the various boxes on the form to convey to the third-party administrator or payer the types of services that were provided to the patient.

Remember...

A key factor for claim submission is determining whether Medicare is the primary insurance or secondary payer. This information affects how the claim form will be completed for reimbursement.

PHARMACIST CARE CLAIM FORMS

The National Community Pharmacist Association (NCPA) developed a popular Pharmacist Care Claim Form (PCCF) with a more specific way of billing for their clinical services (see Figure 15–1). The core of the PCCF consists of six fields of information:

1. Reason for Service
2. Professional Service
3. Result of Service
4. Level of Service
5. Drugs Involved
6. Billing Codes/Professional Fees

The Reason for Service codes are further classified into one of five code groups to better reflect their shared content:

1. Administrative
2. Dosing/Limits
3. Drug Conflict
4. Disease Management
5. Precautionary

PHARMACIST CARE CLAIM FORM

SUBMIT TO
REFERENCE
NUMBER

CERTIFICATION STATEMENT

Subscriber Information

Name _____ Phone _____

Address _____

City _____ State _____ Zip _____

Birthdate _____ Social Security/Subscriber I.D. No. _____

Date of Service _____ Sex __ M __ F __ Employer _____

Employer I.D. _____ Plan No. _____

Group No. _____

Patient

Name _____ Birthdate _____ Sex __ M __ F

Relationship of patient to Subscriber □ Self □ Spouse □ Child □ Other

Full-Time Student □ Yes □ No   If yes, Where? _____

SIGNATURE _____

DATE _____

I. PROBLEMS AND NEEDS	II. ACTIONS AND INTERVENTION	III. RECOMMENDATIONS	IV RESULTS OR OUTCOMES
Drug Product Selection	40 □ Contact Health Care Provider	60 □ Add Drug	80 □ Drug Added
01 □ Drug needed but not prescribed	41 □ Contact Third-Party Payer	61 □ Discontinue Drug	81 □ Drug Discontinued
02 □ Prescribed drug not needed	42 □ Counsel Patient	62 □ Do Not Dispense Drug	82 □ Drug Not Dispensed
03 □ Duplication	43 □ Counsel Patient's Caregiver	63 □ Change Drug	83 □ Drug Changed
04 □ Ease-of-use	44 □ Demonstration	64 □ Change Dose	84 □ Dose Changed
05 □ Efficacy	45 □ Develop Compliance Aid	65 □ Change Dosage Form	85 □ Dosage Form Changed
06 □ Safety	46 □ Education	66 □ Change Route	86 □ Route Changed
07 □ Cost	47 □ Monitor Drug Therapy	67 □ Change Schedule/ Duration	87 □ Schedule/Duration Changed
Regimen	48 □ Refer	68 □ Referral	88 □ Patient Accepted Referral
08 □ Dose	49 □ Consult on Self-Care	69 □ Self-Care	89 □ Patient Accepted Self-Care
09 □ Schedule/Duration	97 □ Other (Specify)	70 □ Continue Without Change	90 □ Recommendation NOT Accepted
10 □ Route		98 □ Other (Specify)	99 □ Other (Specify
11 □ Dosage Form			
Contraindication/Interaction	V. DISCUSSION AND SPECIFIC DRUGS INVOLVED		

Pharmacist Care Information

12 ☐ Age
13 ☐ Disease or condition
14 ☐ Drug
15 ☐ Food
16 ☐ Laboratory
17 ☐ Pregnancy/Nursing
Adverse Effect
18 ☐ Additive Effects
19 ☐ Allergy
20 ☐ Toxicity
Request for Information
21 ☐ Patient
22 ☐ Patient's Caregiver
23 ☐ Health Care provider
24 ☐ Third-Party Payer
Patient Product Misuse
25 ☐ Underuse
26 ☐ Overuse
27 ☐ Abuse
28 ☐ Not Filled or Refilled
29 ☐ Stored Inappropriately
30 ☐ Prescription Clarification
96 ☐ Other (Specify)
* Actual, suspected, or potential drug and health related problems and needs.

Pharmacy Imprint

NAME

ADDRESS

PHONE

NABP NO   SSN/TIN

VI. PROFESSIONAL FEES		
Code	Fee	
Code	Fee	
	Code	Fee
	TOTAL FEE	

I hereby certify that the pharmacist care rendered as indicated has been completed and the fees submitted are the actual fees I have charged and intend to collect for those services.

Signature of Pharmacist

Date _____ License No. _____

FIGURE 15–1   Pharmacist Care Claim Form.

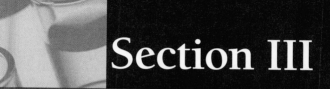

Section III

Drug Classifications and Pharmacologic Actions

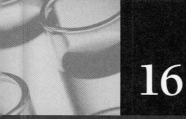

16

Biopharmaceutics

The goal of therapeutics is to achieve a desired beneficial effect with minimal adverse effects. When a drug has been selected for a patient, the physician must determine the dose that most closely achieves this goal.

The pharmacy technician must understand the basics of biopharmaceutical, pharmacokinetic, and pharmacodynamic principles, which collectively describe how a particular medication is prepared, and how it affects the body systems. ■

■ BIOPHARMACEUTICS

Biopharmaceutics is the study of the relationship of the physical and chemical properties of a drug to its effects of:

- Bioavailability
- Pharmacokinetics
- Pharmacodynamics
- Toxicology

BIOAVAILABILITY

Bioavailability is the degree to which a drug releases itself from its dosage form (for example, tablet, capsule, suspension) to become accessible for its intended effect.

PHARMACOKINETICS

Pharmacokinetics is the pharmaceutical science that deals with the absorption, distribution, metabolism, and elimination of drugs and the amount of time each of these processes requires. In many cases, pharmacokinetics can explain the reasons different people react differently to a drug. These differences are determined by the following factors:

- Genetics
- Age
- Gender
- Renal function
- Liver size
- Liver function
- Body temperature
- Nutrition
- Environment
- Drug-drug interactions during drug metabolism
- Smoking

The four processes involved in pharmacokinetics are:

- Absorption
- Distribution
- Metabolism (chemical biotransformation)
- Excretion (elimination)

Figure 16–1 illustrates the processes of pharmacokinetics.

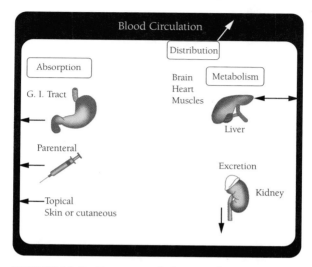

FIGURE 16–1 **Processes of pharmacokinetics.**

Absorption

Absorption is the movement of a drug from its site of administration into the blood. Generally, absorption takes place through the digestive system unless a drug is administered directly into the blood circulation by injection. The absorption of a drug is a key element in determining a drug-dosing regimen. The duration and intensity of a drug's action are directly related to the rate of absorption of the drug. Many factors affect drug absorption, including:

- Solubility of the drug
- Concentration of the drug

- pH of the drug
- Site of absorption
- Absorption surface area
- Blood supply to the site of absorption
- Bioavailability

Remember...

Specific directions must be given, when necessary, to increase absorption of the drug, such as taking it on an empty stomach or taking it when eating food.

The absorption of drugs via the GI tract may be influenced by several factors—physiochemical properties, acidity of the stomach, presence of food in the stomach, dosage, and routes of administration (see Table 16–1).

Distribution

Distribution is the movement of a drug from the blood into the tissues and cells. Most drugs will pass easily from the bloodstream, through the interstitial spaces, and into the target cells. Lipid solubility is important for effective distribution when a drug must pass over the lipid membrane of the cells. Lipid-soluble drugs enter the central nervous system rapidly. Drug administration and its effects on drug action are shown in Figure 16–2.

TABLE 16–1   Factors Affecting Drug Absorption

Factors	Remarks
Physiochemical properties	The rate of absorption of a drug may be affected greatly by the rate at which the drug is made available to the biological fluid at the site of administration.
Acidity of the stomach	Drugs with an acidic pH, such as aspirin, are easily absorbed in the acid environment of the stomach.
Presence of food in the stomach	This factor can have a profound influence on the rate and extent of drug absorption. Food in the stomach decreases the absorption rate of medications, whereas an empty stomach increases the rate.
Dosage	Higher concentrations of drugs can be absorbed much faster than low doses of the drug.
Routes of administration	The choice of the administration route is crucial in determining the suitability of a drug for each patient. IV drugs act rapidly and the process of absorption is bypassed.

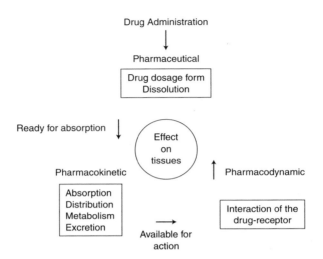

FIGURE 16–2   The effect of drug administration on drug action.

Metabolism

Metabolism is the physical and chemical alteration of the drug in the body. The overwhelming majority of drugs undergo metabolism after they enter the body.

Remember...

The liver is a primary site of drug metabolism. Drugs administered orally are absorbed in the small intestine, and then are metabolized by the liver enzymes before entering the blood circulation. This process is called the first-pass effect.

Excretion

Excretion or elimination of a drug is the removal of waste products of drug metabolism. A drug may be eliminated through:

- Urination
- Respiration (alcohols and anesthetics)
- Perspiration (sweat)
- Defecation (unabsorbed drugs and those secreted in the bile)
- Saliva
- Milk—from a lactating mother

> **Remember...**
>
> The majority of drugs are eliminated through the kidneys. Therefore, good renal function is very important.

> **Remember...**
>
> The processes of pharmacokinetics depend on several factors, such as, age, route of administration, gender, dosage, and conditions of the patient.

PHARMACODYNAMICS

Pharmacodynamics is the study of the interaction of drugs with their sites of action. Pharmacodynamics examines the way drugs bind with their receptors, the concentration required to elicit a response, and the time required for each of these events. In other words, **drug action** is the physiological change in the body or

the response to the drug effect. There are four classifications for drug effects:

- **Stimulation** is caused by an agent that increases
  the activity of a cell, tissue, organ, or the whole
  body. For example, a neurotransmitter such as epinephrine stimulates the heart to beat faster. Drugs
  such as amphetamines and caffeine stimulate the
  central nervous system to increase wakefulness.
- **Depression** is a decrease of some body function or
  activity.
- **Irritation** is caused by an agent that inflames a tissue; this is often a result of drugs applied to the
  skin or mucous membranes.
- **Demulcence** is caused by an agent that soothes
  inflamed or irritated tissue, particularly mucous
  membranes. Most throat lozenges, for example,
  contain a demulcent. A demulcent is most commonly an oil or a syrup.

Drug Action

Drug products are chosen for specific cells because
particular drugs have specific affinities for particular
cells. This specific cell recipient is called a **receptor**.

Various factors are important in determining the
correct drugs for a patient so that it will offer the correct actions. These factors include:

- Drug half-life
- Age
- Gender
- Body weight
- Diurnal body rhythms
- The presence of illnesses

- Psychological factors
- Tolerance
- Drug toxicity
- Drug interactions
- Idiosyncratic reactions

Drug Half-Life

The half-life of a drug is the time it takes for the plasma concentration to be reduced by 50%. This is one of the most common methods used to explain drug actions. The half-life of one drug may be different than that of other drugs. Another method of describing drug action is a graphic depiction of the plasma concentration of the drug versus time (see Figure 16–3).

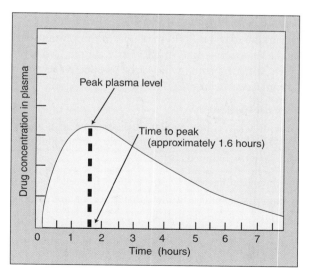

FIGURE 16–3   Plot of drug concentration in plasma versus time after a single oral administration of a drug.

Age

Infants and elderly individuals show the greatest effects of a drug. They are more sensitive to drugs that affect the CNS and are at risk for development of drug toxicity.

Gender

Men and women respond to drugs differently. Some medications pose a risk in pregnant women because of damage to the developing fetus. Drugs remain in women's bodies longer than in men because of higher body fat content.

Body Weight

Basically, the same dosage has less effect in a patient who weighs more, and a greater effect in a patient who weighs less.

Diurnal Body Rhythms

During the day, body rhythms play an important part in the effects of some drugs. For example, sedatives given in the morning will not be as effective as those administered before bedtime.

Presence of Illnesses

Patients with kidney or liver disease may respond to drugs differently because the body cannot detoxify and excrete chemicals properly.

Psychological Factors

A patient's mental attitude can reduce or increase an expected response to a drug.

Tolerance

Development of resistance to the effects of a drug makes it necessary to continually raise doses in an effort to elicit the desired response.

Drug Toxicity

Almost all drugs are capable of producing toxic effects. There is a range between the therapeutic dose of a drug and its toxic dose. This range is measured by the therapeutic index, which is used to explain the safety of a drug.

$$\text{Therapeutic index (TI)} = \frac{LD_{50}}{ED_{50}}$$

As shown, LD_{50} is the lethal dose of a drug that will kill 50% of animals tested, and ED_{50} is the effective dose that produces a specific therapeutic effect in 50% of animals tested. The greater the therapeutic index, the safer a drug is likely to be.

Drug Interactions

Drug interactions are defined as effects that two or more drugs have on each other when used concurrently in the same patient. The following results may be seen:

1. The drugs have no effect on each other's action.

2. The drugs increase each other's effect.

3. The drugs decrease each other's effect.

Idiosyncratic Reactions

Idiosyncratic drug reactions are unexpected, unusual responses to a drug. Unwanted reactions can occur with all medications and should be documented if they occur.

TOXICOLOGY

Toxicology is the study of the poisonous effects of drugs on the body. Toxic effects can occur with all drugs. A single dose of a medication may separate a therapeutic effect from a toxic effect.

17

Human Response to Drug Activity

Drugs are capable of exerting a wide variety of effects in the human body. There are several fundamental pharmacological principles that can be described concerning the action of drugs. However, it should be noted that considerable variation may occur in the response of any two individuals to the same drug and dosage regimen. ▪

FACTORS INFLUENCING THE EFFECTS OF DRUGS

Factors that influence the effects of drugs include:

- Age
- Weight
- Gender
- Genetics
- Psychological factors
- Disease states
- Pregnancy
- Adverse drug reactions
- Drug-drug interactions
- Drug-diet interactions

AGE

The age of a patient may cause the patient to respond to drug activity in different ways. Human life is based on physiological characteristics and has several stages. These stages are as follows:

- Neonate
- Infant
- Child
- Adolescent
- Adult
- Elderly

Neonates and Infants

Neonates and infants usually require smaller doses of a drug than do adults. Immature organ function (such as that of the liver and kidneys) can affect the ability of neonates and infants to metabolize drugs.

Children and Adolescents

Maturation of organ function in older children is improved, but it is important to note that children are able to metabolize certain drugs more rapidly than adults. Their metabolism rate increases between one year and twelve years of age, depending on the child and the drug. Adolescents metabolize drugs almost identically to adults. Some drugs are eliminated through the kidneys faster in children, including the following:

- Ethosuximide
- Theophylline
- Clindamycin
- Valproic acid

Adults

Because of the aging process, adults between the ages of 30 and 70 experience a decrease in many normal body functions. Therefore, drugs metabolize much more slowly.

Elderly

Elderly patients may experience more physiological changes that can influence and significantly affect drug action. They are usually taking multiple drugs, which can potentially react with one another. This might result in an increased potential for adverse reactions. Physiological changes in the elderly include:

- A decrease in metabolism of most drugs
- Changes in gastric pH and GI tract absorption
- Changes in the cardiovascular system (lower cardiac output)
- A decrease in kidney function

WEIGHT

In general, dosages are based on an average weight (150 lb) for both men and women. However, weight is often considered when calculating doses for infants, children, and obese patients.

Remember....

In obese patients, if body fat content is greater than 30% of total body weight, it can significantly change the distribution and renal excretion of a drug.

To calculate the amount of drug based on a child's body weight in kilograms, it is necessary to compare the child's ordered dosage to the recommended safe dosage from a reputable drug resource before administering the medication. During calculation for safe pediatric dosages, convert the child's weight from pounds to kilograms. Multiply mg/kg by the child's weight in kg (for example, 1 kg = 2.2 lbs, or 1 g = 1000 mg).

Remember...

> The dosage per kg may be mg/kg, g/kg, mEq/kg, U/kg, mU/kg, etc.

GENDER

Gender may influence the action of some drugs. Women may require a smaller dose of some drugs than men because of different factors:

- Body fat and muscles
- Weight ratio
- Hormonal fluctuations

GENETICS

Genes are different in each person. Genes can determine the types and amounts of proteins produced in the body. The effect of drug action depends on interaction of proteins in plasma, tissue, and receptor sites.

Remember...

> Patients with genetic abnormalities can respond to drugs differently for absorption, distribution, metabolism, and excretion. The result is that drugs may have no effect at all or provide an adverse (or toxic) effect.

PSYCHOLOGICAL FACTORS

Psychological factors may affect a patient's responses to drug administration. For example, patients who use a placebo may experience therapeutic or adverse effects.

DISEASE STATES

The presence of disease may influence the action of some drugs. Liver and kidney diseases can greatly affect drug response. Drug dosages may be reduced in these conditions.

PREGNANCY

During pregnancy, particularly the latter stages, several physiological changes may occur in women. These changes can result in the following:

- Reduced absorption rate of a drug
- Reduced plasma protein binding
- Increased metabolism of several drugs
- Increased urinary excretion of several drugs

ADVERSE DRUG REACTIONS

Patients may experience one or more adverse drug reactions when they use a drug. Adverse reactions can be defined as undesirable drug effects, and may have different characterizations, as follows:

- Mild, severe, or life-threatening reactions
- Reactions that may occur:
  - After the last dose
  - After several doses
- Unpredictable reactions

Various adverse effects may occur with common or usual doses of drugs, often called side effects, which include:

- Hypersensitivity (allergy)
- Central nervous system effects
  - CNS stimulation
    - Agitation
    - Disorientation
    - Confusion
    - Hallucinations
  - CNS depression
    - Drowsiness
    - Dizziness
    - Sedation
    - Coma
    - Impaired respiration and circulation
- Auditory damage
- Ocular damage
- Hematological effects
  - Bleeding
  - Bone marrow depression
- Hepatotoxicity
- Nephrotoxicity
- Gastrointestinal effects
  - Nausea, vomiting

- Constipation
- Diarrhea
- Anorexia
- Peptic ulcer
- Colitis
- Teratogenicity (causing abnormal fetal development when given to pregnant women)
- Toxicity
- Carcinogenicity

The following commonly used drugs may cause hepatotoxicity:

- Acetaminophen
- Aspirin
- Chlorpromazine
- Halothane
- Isoniazid
- Methotrexate
- Nitrofurantoin
- Phenytoin

Remember...

Allergic reactions can occur within minutes or weeks of drug administration. Anaphylactic shock occurs within minutes.

Remember...

Anaphylactic shock is life-threatening. Immediate emergency treatment is required. To treat anaphylactic shock, the following drugs must be administered: epinephrine, antihistamines, or bronchodilators.

DRUG INTERACTIONS

Drug interactions refer to the effects that occur when the actions of one drug are affected by another drug. There are many different types of drug interactions in which the mechanism of actions include:

- Interference during GI absorption
- Interference with plasma protein binding
- Drug metabolism
- Drug excretion

To understand drug-drug interactions, the pharmacy technician must be familiar with the following terms:

- **Additive effects:** Effects wherein two or more substances used in combination produce a total effect that is the same as the sum of the individual effects
- **Antidote:** Drug or substance given to stop a toxic effect
- **Antagonism:** Reduction of one drug's effect by another drug
- **Displacement:** A change in which one element, radical, or molecule is replaced by another, or in which one element exchanges electric charges with another by reduction or oxidation
- **Induction:** The period of time between the beginning of administration of a general anesthetic and

the point at which the patient has achieved the desired level of unconsciousness

- **Inhibition:** The arrest of a process normally performed by a molecule of a drug

- **Potentiation:** An interaction between two drugs that causes an effect greater than would have been expected from the additive properties of the drugs involved. (For example, alcohol potentiates the sedating effects of the tranquilizer diazepam when the two drugs are ingested at the same time.)

- **Synergism:** A combined action of two or more agents that produces an effect greater than would have been expected from the two agents acting separately

- **Summation:** Combining drugs to achieve the expected effect of each drug

DRUG-DIET INTERACTIONS

The influence of nutrition on the metabolism of drugs depends on microsomal enzyme activity by the presence of certain vitamins and minerals. Deficiencies of the following vitamins, minerals, and foods can result in ineffective metabolism:

- Vitamins A, B, and B_2
- The minerals copper, zinc, or calcium
- Proteins
- Essential fatty acids

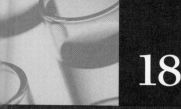

18

Drug Effects and Drug Classifications

Pharmacology can be defined as the study of substances that interact with living systems through chemical processes that alter the body's function. Drug effects on different systems of the body will be summarized in this chapter. ∎

CENTRAL NERVOUS SYSTEM

Drug classifications affecting the central nervous system (CNS) include:

- Sedatives, hypnotics, and antianxiety drugs
- Anticonvulsants
- Antiparkinson drugs
- Antidepressants
- Antipsychotics
- Narcotic analgesics
- Anesthetics

SEDATIVES, HYPNOTICS, AND ANTIANXIETY DRUGS

Sedatives and hypnotic drugs are used to treat anxiety and sleep disorders. Sedatives can reduce anxiety. Hypnotic drugs are used to produce sleep or drowsiness. Table 18–1 summarizes the most common drugs used for anxiety.

Remember...

Since the development of the benzodiazepines, barbiturates are rarely used for anxiety. Barbiturates have a higher risk of adverse effects and toxicity than benzodiazepines.

TABLE 18–1   Most Common Sedatives and Hypnotics

Generic Name	Trade Name	Route of Administration	Average Adult Dosage
Benzodiazepines			
alprazolam	Xanax	PO	0.25–0.5 mg tid, max: 4 mg/d

(continued)

chlordiazepoxide	Librium	PO, IM, IV	PO: 5–10 mg tid–qid; IM/IV: 50–100 mg 1 h before surgery
clorazepate dipotassium	Tranxene	PO	30 mg followed by 30–60 mg in div. doses
diazepam	Valium	PO, IM, IV, Rectal	PO: 2–10 mg bid–qid or 15–30 mg/d sustained release; IV/IM: 2–10 mg, repeat if needed in 3–4 h
estazolam	Prosom	PO	1 mg h.s., may increase up to 2 mg if necessary
flurazepam hydrochloride	Dalmane	PO	15–30 mg h.s.
lorazepam	Ativan	PO, IM, IV	PO: 2–6 mg/d in div. doses; IM: 2–4 mg (0.05 mg/kg) at least 2 h before surgery; IV: 0.044 mg/kg up to 2 mg 15–20 min before surgery
oxazepam	Serax	PO	10–30 mg tid–qid
quazepam	Doral	PO	7.5–15 mg h.s.

(continued)

triazolam	Halcion	PO	0.125–0.25 mg h.s. (max: 0.5 mg/d)
Nonbenzodiazepines			
buspirone hydrochloride	BuSpar	PO	7.5–15 mg/d in div. doses
chloral hydrate	Aquachloral	PO, Rectal	PO/PR Sedative: 250 mg tid pc; PO/PR Hypnotic: 500 mg–1 g, 15–30 min before h.s. or 30 min before surgery
phenobarbital sodium	Luminal	PO, IM, IV	PO: 100–300 mg/d; IV/IM: 200–600 mg up to 20 mg/kg
secobarbital sodium	Seconal	PO	100–300 mg/d in 3 div. doses
zaleplon	Sonata	PO	10 mg h.s. (max: 20 mg h.s.)
zolpidem tartrate	Ambien	PO	5–10 mg h.s., limited to 7–10 d

ANTICONVULSANTS

Epilepsy is a group of disorders that are characterized by hyperexcitability within the CNS. **Seizure** is a term for all epileptic events, whereas **convulsion** refers to abnormal motor movements. Antiepileptic drugs prevent or stop a convulsive seizure. Classifications of epileptic events are shown in Table 18–2.

TABLE 18–2   Epilepsy Classifications

I. Focal or Partial Seizures	II. Generalized Seizures
A. Simple seizures	A. Nonconvulsive
	1. Absence or petit mal seizures
B. Complex partial	B. Convulsive seizures
	1. Tonic/clonic or grand mal seizures
	2. Tonic/psychomotor seizures
	3. Status epilepticus

The major drugs used to control seizures are phenytoin, carbamazepine, and valproic acid. Other medications are listed in Table 18–3.

TABLE 18–3 Anticonvulsants

Generic Name	Trade Name	Route of Administration	Average Adult Dosage
carbamazepine	Tegretol, Tegretol XR	PO	200 mg bid, gradually increased to 800–1200 mg/d in 3–4 div. doses. Tegretol XR dosed bid
clonazepam	Klonopin	PO	1.5 mg/d in div. doses, increase by 0.5–1 mg q3d until seizures are controlled
diazepam	Valium	PO, IM, IV	PO: 2–10 mg bid–qid or 15–30 mg/d sustained release; IV/IM: 2–10 mg, repeat if needed in 3–4 h
ethosuximide	Zarontin	PO	250 mg bid, may increase q4–7d prm (max: 1.5 g/d)

(continued)

felbamate	Felbatol	PO	Initiate with 1200 mg/d in 3–4 div. doses, may increase by 600 mg/d q2wk (max: 3600 mg/d)
fosphenytoin sodium	Cerebyx	IM, IV	15–20 mg/kg
gabapentin	Neurontin	PO	Initiate with 300 mg on day 1, 300 mg bid on day 2, 300 mg tid on day 3, increase over a week to initial total dose of 400 mg tid (1200 mg/d), may increase to 1800–2400 mg/d depending on response (most receive 900–1800 mg/d in 3 div. doses) 400 mg tid (1200 mg/d)
lamotrigine	Lamictal	PO	Start with 25 mg qod for 2wks, then 25 mg qd for 2wks, may titrate up to 150 mg/d in 2 div. doses
levetiracetam	Keppra	PO	500 mg bid, may increase by 500 mg bid q2wks

(continued)

lorazepam	Ativan	IV for status epilepticus	4 mg injected slowly at 2 mg/min, may repeat dose once if inadequate response after 10 min
phenytoin	Dilantin	PO, IV	PO: 15–18 mg/kg or 1g loading dose, then 300 mg/d in 1–3 div. doses; IV: 15–18 mg/kg or 1g loading dose, then 100 mg tid
primidone	Mysoline	PO	250 mg/d, increased 250 mg/wk
tiagabine hydrochloride	Gabitril	PO	Start with 4 mg qd, may increase dose by 4–8 mg/d q wk
topiramate	Topamax	PO	Initiate with 25 mg bid, increase by 50 mg/wk to efficacy
valproic acid	Depakene	PO, IV	15 mg/kg/d in div. doses when total daily dose >250 mg, increase at 1 wk intervals by 5–10 mg/kg/d until seizures are controlled

(continued)

| zonisamide | Zonegran | PO | Start at 100 mg q.d., may increase after 2wks to 200 mg/d, may increase q2wks if necessary (max: 400 mg/d in 1–2 div.doses) |

ANTIPARKINSON DRUGS

Parkinson's disease is characterized by:

- Resting tremor
- Resistance to passive movement
- Akinesia
- Loss of postural reflexes
- Behavioral manifestations

Table 18–4 shows some drugs for Parkinson's disease.

TABLE 18–4   Antiparkinson Drugs

Generic Name	Trade Name	Route of Administration	Average Adult Dosage
amantadine hydrochloride	Symmetrel	PO	100 mg 1–2 times/d, start with 100 mg/d if patient is on other anti-Parkinsonism medications
benztropine mesylate	Cogentin	PO	0.5–1 mg/d, may gradually increase as needed up to 6 mg/d
bromocriptine mesylate	Parlodel	PO	1.25–2.5 mg/d (max: 100 mg/d in div. doses)
carbidopa/levodopa	Sinemet	PO	(if not currently receiving levodopa): 1 tablet containing 10 mg carbidopa/100 mg levodopa or 25 mg carbidopa/100 mg levodopa tid, increased by 1 tablet qd–qod up to 6 tablets/d; (if currently receiving

(continued)

			levodopa): 1 tablet of the 25/250 mixture tid–qid, adjusted by $\frac{1}{2}$–1 tablet as needed up to 8 tablets/d (start at 20–25% of initial dose of levodopa)
entacapone	Comtan	PO	200 mg administered with each dose of levodopa/carbidopa up to 8 times/d
levodopa	Dopar, Larodopa	PO	500 mg to 1 g daily in 2 or more equally div. doses, may be increased by 100–750 mg q3–7d (max: 8g/d); used in combination with carbidopa, decrease levodopa dose by 75–80%
pramipexole	Mirapex	PO	Start with 0.125 mg tid times 1 wk, then 0.25 mg tid times 1 wk, continue to increase by 0.25 mg/dose tid q wk to a target dose of 1.5 mg tid
ropinirole hydrochloride	Requip	PO	Start with 0.25 mg tid, may titrate up by 0.25 mg/dose tid q wk to a target dose of

(continued)

| trihexyphenidyl hydrochloride | Trihexy | PO | 1 mg tid; if response is still not satisfactory; may continue to increase by 1.5 mg/d q wk to a dose of 9 mg/d, and then by less than or equal to 3 mg/d weekly (max: 24 mg/d) |
| | | | 1 mg day 1, 2 mg day 2, then increase by 2 mg q3–5d up to 6–10 mg/d in 3 or more div. doses (max: 15 mg/d) |

ANTIDEPRESSANTS

Depression is one of the most common psychiatric disorders in the United States. It is characterized by:

- Feelings of intense sadness
- Feelings of helplessness
- Feelings of worthlessness
- Impaired functioning
- Inability to experience pleasure in activities
- Loss of energy
- Changes in sleep habits
- Sudden weight gain or loss

Drugs used to treat depression are shown in Table 18–5.

TABLE 18-5   Drugs Used to Treat Depression

Generic Name	Trade Name	Route of Administration	Average Adult Dosage
Tricyclic Antidepressants			
amitriptyline hydrochloride	Elavil, Endep	PO, IM	PO: 75–100 mg/d, may gradually increase to 150–300 mg/d (use lower doses in outpatients); IM: 20–30 mg qid until patient can take PO
clomipramine hydrochloride	Anafranil	PO	50–150 mg/d in single or div. doses
desipramine hydrochloride	Norpramin	PO	75–100 mg/d at bedtime or in div. doses, may gradually increase to 150–300 mg/d (use lower doses in older adult patients)

(continued)

doxepin hydrochloride	Sinequan, Adapin	PO	30–150 mg/d h.s. or in div. doses, may gradually increase to 300 mg/d (use lower doses in older adult patients)
imipramine hydrochloride	Tofranil	PO, IM	PO: 75–100 mg/d (max: 300 mg/d) in 1 or more div. doses; IM: 50–100 mg/d in div. doses
nortriptyline hydrochloride	Aventyl, Pamelor	PO	25 mg tid–qid gradually increased to 100–150 mg/d
Second-Generation Cyclic Antidepressants			
bupropion hydrochloride	Wellbutrin, Wellbutrin SR, Zyban	PO	75–100 mg tid, start with 75 mg tid, or 100 mg (SR) bid, or 150 mg (XL) qd, and increase dose q3d to 300 mg/d; doses >450 mg/d are associated with an increased risk of adverse reactions including seizures
mirtazapine	Remeron	PO	15 mg/d in single dose h.s., may increase q1–2wks (max: 45 mg/d)

(continued)

nefazodone	Serzone	PO	50–100 mg bid, may need to increase up to 300–600 mg/d in 2–3 div. doses
trazodone hydrochloride	Desyrel	PO	150 mg/d in div. doses, may increase by 50 mg/d q3–4d (max: 400–600 mg/d)
Monoamine Oxidase Inhibitors			
phenelzine sulfate	Nardil	PO	15 mg tid; rapidly increase to at least 60 mg/d, may need up to 90 mg/d
Selective Serotonin Reuptake Inhibitors			
citalopram hydrobromide	Celexa	PO	Start at 20 mg qd, may increase to 40 mg qd if needed
fluoxetine hydrochloride	Prozac	PO	20 mg/d in a.m., may increase by 20 mg/d at weekly intervals (max: 80 mg/d); 20 mg/d in a.m.; when stable may switch to 90 mg sustained-release capsule q wk (max: 90 mg/wk)

(continued)

fluvoxamine	Luvox	PO	Start with 50 mg qd, may increase slowly up to 300 mg/d given qhs or div. bid
paroxetine	Paxil	PO	10–50 mg/d (max: 80 mg/d); 25 mg sustained-release qd in a.m., may increase by 12.5 mg (max: 62.5 mg/d); use lower starting doses for patients with renal or hepatic insufficiency and geriatric patients
sertraline hydrochloride	Zoloft	PO	Begin with 50 mg/d, gradually increase every few weeks according to response (range: 50–200 mg)
venlafaxine	Effexor	PO	25–125 tid
Medications for Bipolar Disorder			
lithium carbonate	Eskalith, Lithobid	PO	Loading: 600 mg tid or 900 mg sustained-release bid or 30 mL (48 mEq) of solution tid; Maintenance: 300 mg tid–qid or 15–20 mL (24–32 mEq) solution in 2–4 div. doses (max: 2.4 g/d)

(continued)

lithium citrate	Cibalith-S (syrup)	PO	(same as lithium carbonate above)
sodium valproate	Depakene, Depakote	PO	250 mg tid (max: 60 mg/kg/d)

ANTIPSYCHOTICS

Psychosis is a mental disorder, such as schizophrenia, in which a person's capacity to recognize reality is distorted. Psychosis is characterized by the following symptoms:

- Hallucinations (hearing or observing things that are not real)
- Delusions (fixed beliefs that are false)

Antipsychotics can be classified as conventional and atypical agents. Drugs used to treat psychosis are shown in Table 18–6.

Remember...

Conventional antipsychotics are thought to act by blocking the action of the neurotransmitter dopamine. Atypical agents appear to block not only dopamine, but also serotonin.

TABLE 18–6 Antipsychotics

Generic Name	Trade Name	Route of Administration	Average Adult Dosage
Conventional Antipsychotics			
High-Potency			
fluphenazine hydrochloride	Prolixin	PO, IM, SC	PO: 0.5–10 mg/d in 1–4 div. doses (max: 20 mg/d); IM/SC HCl: 2.5–10 mg/d div. doses q6–8h (max: 10 mg/d); Decanoate: 12.5–25 mg q1–4wks; Enanthate: 25 mg q2wks

(continued)

haloperidol	Haldol	PO, IM	PO: 0.2–5 mg bid-tid; IM: 2–5 mg repeated q4h prn; Decanoate: 50–100 mg q4wks
thiothixene hydrochloride	Navane	PO, IM	PO: 2 mg tid, may increase up to 15 mg/d as needed or tolerated (max: 60 mg/d); IM: 4 mg bid-qid (max: 30 mg/d)
trifluoperazine hydrochloride	Stelazine	PO, IM	PO: 1–2 mg bid, may increase up to 20 mg/d in hospitalized patients; IM: 1–2 mg q4–6h (max: 10 mg/d)
Intermediate-Potency			
loxapine succinate	Loxitane	PO, IM	PO: Start with 10 mg bid and rapidly increase to maintenance levels of 60–100 mg/d in 2–4 div. doses (max: 250 mg/d); IM: 12.5–50 mg q4–6h

(continued)

perphenazine	Trilafon	PO, IM, IV	PO: 4–16 mg bid–qid; 8–32 mg sustained release bid (max: 64 mg/d); IM: 5 mg q6h (max: 15–30 mg/d); IV: Dilute to 0.5 mg/mL in NS, administer at not more than 1 mg q1–2 min or 5 mg by slow infusion
Low-Potency			
chlorpromazine hydrochloride	Thorazine	PO, IM, IV	PO: 25–100 mg tid–qid, may need up to 1000 mg/d; IM/IV: 25–50 mg up to 600 mg q4–6h
thioridazine hydrochloride	Mellaril	PO	50–100 mg tid, may increase up to 800 mg/d as needed or tolerated
Atypical Antipsychotics			
aripiprazole	Abilify	PO	10–15 mg/d, may increase at 2 wk intervals to max of 30 mg/d prn

(continued)

clozapine	Clozaril	PO	Initiate at 25–50 mg/d and titrate to a target dose of 350–450 mg/d in 3 div. doses at 2 wk intervals; increase prn (max: 900 mg/d)
olanzapine	Zyprexa	PO	Start with 5–10 mg/d, may increase by 2.5–5 mg q wk until desired response (usual range 10–15 mg/d, max: 20 mg/d)
quetiapine fumarate	Seroquel	PO	Initiate with 25 mg bid, may increase by 25–50 mg bid–tid on 2nd or 3rd day as tolerated to a target dose of 300–400 mg/d div. doses bid–tid, may adjust dose by 25–50 mg bid qd prn (max: 800 mg/d)
risperidone	Risperdal	PO, IM	PO: 1–6 mg bid, start with 1 mg bid, increase by 1 mg bid to an initial target dose of 3 mg bid (max: 8 mg/d); IM: 25 mg once q2wks (max: 50 mg)

(continued)

| | | PO: Start with 20 mg bid w/food, may increase q2d up to 80 mg bid prn; IM: 10 mg q2h or 20 mg q4h up to max of 40 mg/d |

| ziprasidone hydrochloride | Geodon | PO, IM |

NARCOTIC ANALGESICS

Narcotic analgesics are also referred to as **opioids**, which is the general term for drugs with morphine-like activity that reduce pain, and induce tolerance and physical dependence. Drugs made from opium (such as morphine and heroin) are referred to as **opiates**. Table 18–7 shows the most common narcotic analgesics.

TABLE 18–7   Narcotic Analgesics

Generic Name	Trade Name	Route of Administration	Average Adult Dosage
codeine	None	PO, IM, SC	15–60 mg qid

(continued)

fentanyl citrate	Duragesic, Sublimaze	PO, IM, Transdermal	PO: Suck on 400-mcg lozenge until sedated; IM(premedication): 50–100 mcg 30–60 min before surgery; IM(postop pain): 50–100 mcg q1–2h prn; Transdermal: Individualize and regularly reasses doses of transdermal fentanyl; for patient not already receiving an opioid, initial dose is 25 mcg/h patch q3d; for patients already on opioids, see package insert for conversions
hydrocodone bitartrate	Hycodan, Robidone A	PO	5–10 mg q4–6h prn (max: 15 mg/dose)
hydromorphone hydrochloride	Dilaudid, Palladone	PO, IM, IV, Rectal, SC	PO/IM/IV/SC: 1–4 mg q4–6h prn; extended release: 12–32 mg q24h; Rectal: 3 mg q4–6h
meperidine hydrochloride	Demerol	PO, IM, IV, SC	50–150 mg q3–4h prn
methadone hydrochloride	Dolophine, Methadone	PO, IM, SC	2.5–10 mg q3–4h prn

(continued)

morphine sulfate	Avinza, Duramorph	PO, IM, IV, SC, Rectal	PO: 10–30 mg q4h prn or 15–30 mg sustained-release q8–12h; Avinza: dose q24h; IV: 2.5–15 mg q4h or 0.8–10 mg/h by continuous infusion, may increase prn to control pain or 5–10 mg epidurally q24h; IM/SC: 5–20 mg q4h; PR: 10–20 mg q4h prn
pentazocine hydrochloride	Talwin, Talwin NX	PO, IM, IV, SC	PO: 50–100 mg q3–4h (max: 600 mg/d); IM/IV/SC: 30 mg q3–4h (max: 360 mg/d)
propoxyphene hydrochloride or napsylate	Darvon-N	PO	65 mg HCl or 100 mg napsylate q4h prn

ANESTHETICS

Anesthesia, literally, is the unique condition of reversible unconsciousness or a loss of sensation. Anesthesia is characterized by four reversible actions:

- Unconsciousness
- Analgesia
- Immobility
- Amnesia

There are four stages of general anesthesia (see Table 18–8).

TABLE 18–8 Stages of Anesthesia

Stages	Characterized By
Stage I	Analgesia Euphoria Perceptual distortions Amnesia
Stage II	Delirium Hypertension Tachycardia
Stage III	Surgical anesthesia
Stage IV	Medullary depression begins with cessation of respiration and circulatory collapse

There are two classes of anesthetic agents:

- Local anesthetics
- General anesthetics

Examples of local anesthetics are shown in Table 18–9 and general anesthetics that are currently in use are shown in Table 18–10.

TABLE 18–9 Local Anesthetics

Generic Name	Trade Name	Route of Administration	Average Adult Dosage
Amides			
bupivacaine hydrochloride	Marcaine, Sensorcaine	IM (local infiltration, sympathetic block, lumbar epidural, caudal block, peripheral nerve block, retrobulbar block)	0.25% to 0.75% solutions depending on how administered

(continued)

etidocaine hydrochloride	Duranest	IM (percutaneous, peripheral nerve block-caudal, central neural block)	0.5%–1.5% solution (max: 300 mg or 400 mg if given with epinephrine)
lidocaine hydrochloride	Xylocaine, Anestacon	Caudal, Epidural, Infiltration, Nerve Block, Saddle Block, Spinal, Topical (jelly, ointment, cream, or solution)	0.5–2% solution (infil., nerve block, epid., caudal); Spinal: 5% w/glucose; S.B.: 1.5% w/dextrose; Topical: 2.5–5%
Esters			
benzocaine	Americaine, Anbesol	Topical	Lowest effective dose
chloroprocaine hydrochloride	Nesacaine	Caudal, Epidural, Infiltration, Nerve Block	Infil & N.B.: 1–2% solution, max of 800 mg w/o epinephrine, 1 g w/epinephrine; Caudal & Epidural: 2–3% solution, max of 800 mg w/o epinephrine, 1 g w/epinephrine

(continued)

Drug	Trade name	Route	Dose
cocaine (and cocaine hydrochloride)	None	Topical	1–10% solution (use >4% solution with caution), max single dose: 1 mg/kg
dibucaine	Nupercainal	Topical	Apply prn: max 1 oz (28 g/d)
procaine hydrochloride	Novocain	SC	10% solution diluted with NS at 1 mL/5 sec
tetracaine hydrochloride	Pontocaine	Spinal, Topical	Spinal: 1% solution diluted w/equal volume of 10% dextrose in subarachnoid space; Topical: before procedure, 1–2 drops of 0.5% solution or 1.25–2.5 cm ointment in lower conjunctival fornix, or 0.5% solution or ointment to nose or throat

TABLE 18–10 Currently Used General Anesthetics

Generic Name	Trade Name	Route of Administration	Average Adult Dosage
diazepam (a benzodiazepine)	Valium	IV, IM	5–10 mg, repeat if needed in 2–4 h
methohexital sodium	Brevital Sodium	IV	5–12 mL of 1% solution (50–120 mg) at a rate of 1 mL (5 mg) q5min, then 2–4 mL (20–40 mg) q4–7 min prn
midazolam hydrochloride (a benzodiazepine)	Versed	IV	Premedicated: 0.15–0.25 mg/kg over 20–30 s, allow 2 min for effect; Nonpremedicated: 0.3–0.35 mg/kg over 20–30 s, allow 2 min for effect
propofol (a benzodiazepine)	Diprivan	IV	Induction: 2–2.5 mg/kg q10 s until induction onset; Maint: 100–200 mcg/kg/min
thiopental sodium (a barbiturate)	Pentothal	IV	IV test dose: 25–75 mg, then 50–75 mg at 20–40 s intervals; an additional 50 mg may be given prn

ENDOCRINE SYSTEM

The endocrine system consists of specialized cell clusters, glands, hormones, and target tissues. Endocrine drugs are used to treat deficiencies or excesses of specific hormones, or nonendocrine diseases.

DRUGS TO CONTROL THYROID DISEASES

Diseases of the thyroid gland include:

- Hypothyroidism
- Hyperthyroidism
- Overproduction of thyroid hormone

Selected medications used as drugs for the thyroid gland are shown in Table 18–11.

TABLE 18–11 Selected Medications for Thyroid Gland Conditions

Generic Name	Trade Name	Route of Administration	Average Adult Dosage
Antithyroid Preparations			
potassium iodide	Pima, SSKI	PO	50–250 mg tid for 10–14 d before surgery
methimazole	Tapazole	PO	5–15 mg q8h
Calcitonin			
calcitonin (salmon)	Calcimar; Miacalcin	IM, SC	100 IU/d, may increase to 50–100 IU/d or qod
Natural Thyroid Replacement			
(dessicated) thyroid (T₃ and T₄)	Armour Thyroid, Thyrar	PO	60 mg/d, may increase q30d to 60–180 mg/d

(continued)

Synthetic Thyroid Replacement

levothyroxine sodium (thyroxine, T_4)	Levothroid, Synthroid	PO, IV	PO: 25–50 mcg/d, gradually increased by 50–100 mcg q1–4wks to usual dose of 100–400 mcg/d; IV: $\frac{1}{2}$ of usual PO dose
liothyronine sodium (triiodothyronine, T_3)	Cytomel, Triostat	PO	25–75 mcg/d
liotrix (T_3; T_4)	Euthroid, Thyrolar	PO	12.5–30 mcg/d, gradually increase to desired response

DRUGS TO CONTROL DIABETES

The two general classifications for diabetes mellitus include:

- Type I, or insulin-dependent diabetes mellitus (IDDM)
- Type II, or non-insulin-dependent diabetes mellitus (NIDDM)

Remember...

Type I diabetes is characterized by a lack of insulin production from the pancreas, and must be treated with insulin.

Remember...

Type II diabetes may be characterized by either decreased production of insulin, or normal amounts of insulin with abnormal sensitivity of the tissues to the insulin that is present.

Insulin can be given only by injection either subcutaneously or intravenously. Table 18–12 shows a list of different types of insulin.

Remember...

Only regular insulin can be administered intravenously. Insulin doses are measured in units.

TABLE 18–12 Types of Insulin

Insulin Type	Onset of Action	Duration of Action
Rapid-Acting		
Lispro (Aspart)	5–15 minutes	3–4 hours
Short-Acting		
Regular	30–60 minutes	4–6 hours
Intermediate-Acting		
NPH	2–4 hours	10–16 hours
Lente	3–4 hours	12–18 hours
Long-Acting		
Ultralente	6–10 hours	18–20 hours
Glargine	4 hours	24 hours (no peak)

Oral hypoglycemics are used to lower blood sugar in Type II diabetes. Table 18–13 shows a list of oral hypoglycemics.

TABLE 18–13 Oral Hypoglycemic Drugs

Generic Name	Trade Name	Average Adult Dosage	Comments
Sulfonylureas			
First Generation			Long-acting agents
chlorpropamide	Diabinese	Initial: 100–250 mg/d w/breakfast, adjust by 50–125 mg/d q3–5d until glycemic control is achieved, up to 750 mg/d	
tolbutamide	Orinase	250 mg to 3 g/d in 1–2 div. doses	
Second Generation			Used in combinations or as monotherapy
glimepiride	Amaryl	Start with 1–2 mg/d w/breakfast or first main	

(continued)

(continued)

glipizide	Glucotrol, Glucotrol XL	meal, may increase to usual maint dose of 1–4 mg/d (max: 8 mg/d) 2.5–5 mg/d 30 min before breakfast, may increase by 2.5–5 mg q1–2wks; >15 mg/d in div. doses 30 min before a.m. and p.m. meal (max: 40 mg/d); 5–10 mg sustained release tablets once/d
glyburide	DiaBeta, Glynase, Micronase	1.25–5 mg/d w/breakfast, may increase by 2.5–5 mg q1–2wks; >15 mg/d should be given in div. doses w/a.m. and p.m. meal (max: 20 mg/d); micronized: 1.5–3 mg/d (max: 12 mg/d)

Meglitinides (secretogogues)

nateglinide	Starlix	60–120 mg tid 1–30 min prior to meals	May be used as monotherapy or with metformin
repaglinide	Prandin	Initial: 0.5 mg 15–30 min ac; init dose for patients previously using glucose-lowering agents: 1–2 mg 15–30 min ac (2–4 doses/d depending on meal pattern; max: 16 mg/d); dosage range: 0.5–4 mg 15–30 min ac	

Biguanides

metformin hydrochloride	Glucophage, Glucophage XR	Start w/500 mg qd–tid or 850 mg qd–bid w/meals,	One-a-day formulation that helps with G.I. discomfort

(continued)

		may increase by 500–850 mg/d q1–3wks (max: 2550 mg/d); or start w/500 mg sustained release w/p.m. meal, may increase by 500 mg/d at p.m. meal q wk (max: 2000 mg/d)	
Thiazolidinediones (Glitazones)			Monitoring of liver enzymes
pioglitazone hydrochloride	Actos	15–30 mg once/d (max: 45 mg qd)	
rosiglitazone maleate	Avandia	Start at 4 mg qd or 2 mg bid, may increase after 12 w (max: 8 mg/d in 1–2 div. doses)	

(continued)

Alpha-Glucosidase Inhibitors

		Taken with meals
acarbose	Precose	Initiate w/25 mg qd–tid w/meals, may increase q4–8w up to 50–100 mg tid w/meals (max: 150 mg/d for less than or equal to 60 kg, 300 mg/d for more than 60 kg)
miglitol	Glyset	25 mg tid at start of each meal, may increase after 4–8 w to 50 mg tid (max: 100 mg tid)

Combination Agents

These new combinations were developed to increase the compliance of patients.

(continued)

glipizide/metformin	Metoglip	--------
glyburide/metformin	Glucovance	
metforminrosiglitazone/metformin	Avandamet	

ORAL CONTRACEPTIVES

Natural estrogenic hormones are produced by the ovaries and placenta. Progesterone is secreted primarily by the ovarian cells. A female's menstrual cycle is controlled by both estrogen and progesterone. Manipulating estrogen and progesterone (a popular method of contraception) can prevent pregnancy.

Oral contraceptives are the most commonly used drugs to prevent pregnancy. Oral contraceptives include:

1. Estrogen and progestin combinations
2. Progestin-only preparations

Table 18–14 shows a list of the most commonly used contraceptive agents.

TABLE 18–14 The Most Commonly Used Contraceptive Agents

Generic Name	Trade Name	Route of Administration	Average Adult Dosage
Monophasic Agents			
estrogen/progestin	Alesse-28, Necon 1/35, Ortho-Novum 1/35	PO	1 active tablet daily for 21d, then placebo tablet or no tablets for 7 d, repeat cycle
estinyl estradiol/desogestrel	Desogen, Ortho-Cept	PO	
estinyl estradiol/ethynodiol diacetate	Demulen	PO	
estinyl estradiol/levonorgestrel	Alesse, Levlen, Nordette	PO	
estinyl estradiol/norgestrel	Lo/Ovral, Ovral	PO	
ethinyl estradiol/drospirenone	Yasmin	PO	

(continued)

ethinyl estradiol/norelgestromin	Ortho Evra	Transdermal patch
ethinyl estradiol/norethindrone (in various strengths)	Loestrin, Modicon, Norinyl, Ortho-Novum, OvconGenora 1/50,	PO
mestranol/norethindrone	Norethrin, Norinyl	PO
Biphasic Agents		
ethinyl estradiol/norethindrone	Ortho-Novum 10/11	PO
Triphasic Agents		
ethinyl estradiol/levonorgestrel	Tri-Levlen, Triphasil	PO
ethinyl estradiol/norethindrone	Ortho-Novum 7/7/7, Tri-Norinyl	PO
ethinyl estradiol/norgestimate	Ortho Tri-Cyclen	PO
Estrophasic Agents		
ethinyl estradiol/norethindrone	Estrostep	PO

(continued)

Progestin-Only Agents

norethindrone	Micronor, Nor-Q.D.	PO	0.35 mg/d starting on day 1 of menstrual flow, then continuing indefinitely
norgestrel	Ovrette	PO	0.075 mg/d starting on day 1 of menstrual flow, then continuing indefinitely

Long-Acting Agents

intrauterine progesterone contraceptive system	Progestasert	IM, IUD	
levonorgestrel	Mirena	IUD	Insert device on 7th day of menstrual cycle, may leave in place up to 5 years

(continued)

| medroxyprogesterone acetate | Depo-Provera | IM | 100 mg q3 months |
| medroxyprogesterone acetate/ estradiol cypionate | Lunelle | IM | 0.5 mL q 28 days |

CARDIOVASCULAR SYSTEM

Cardiovascular disorders are among the most common causes of death in the United States. These disorders include:

- Angina pectoris
- Hypertension
- Myocardial infarction
- Hyperlipidemia

ANTIANGINA DRUG THERAPY

Angina pectoris is a sharp pain usually felt in the chest or arm. The pain occurs when the heart does not receive a sufficient amount of oxygen to support its workload. Anginal pain most commonly follows exertion.

There are three groups of medications that can help achieve the treatment goals for angina pectoris:

1. Nitrates
2. β-Adrenergic blockers
3. Calcium channel blockers

Commonly used antianginal drugs are listed in Table 18–15.

TABLE 18-15 Commonly Used Antianginal Drugs

Generic Name	Trade Name	Route of Administration	Average Adult Dosage
Nitrates			
isosorbide dinitrate	Isordil, Sorbitrate	PO	Sublingual tablet 2.5–10 mg q2–3h prn; chewable tablet 5–30 mg chewed prn for relief
isosorbide mononitrate	Imdur	PO	30–60 mg q a.m., may increase up to 120 mg once/d after

(continued)

nitroglycerin	Nitro-Bid, Nitrol	PO, Topical	several days if needed (max: dose 240 mg)
			PO: 1.3–9 mg q8–12h; Topical: 1.5–5 cm ($\frac{1}{2}$–2 in) of ointment q4–6h
	Nitrodisc, Nitro-Dur	Transdermal patch	q24h, or leave on for 10–12 h, then remove and have a 10–12 h nitrate-free interval
	Nitrostat, Nitrolingual	Sublingual (SL)	PO: 1.3–9 mg q8–12h; SL: 1–2 sprays (0.4–0.8 mg) or a 0.3–0.6 mg tablet q3–5 min prn (max: 3 doses in 15 min)
	Nitrostat IV, Tridil	IV	Start with 5 mcg/min and titrated q3–5min until desired response
β-Adrenergic Blockers			
acebutolol	Sectral Tenormin		300–400 mg tid

(continued)

atenolol			25–50 mg/d, may increase to 100 mg/d; IV: 5 mg q5min × 2 doses, then switch to PO
metoprolol	Lopressor, Toprol XL		100 mg/d in 2 div. doses, may increase weekly up to 100–400 mg/d
nadolol	Corgard		40 mg once/d, may increase up to 240–320 mg/d in 1–2 div. doses
propranolol hydrochloride	Inderal		10–20 mg bid–tid, may need 160–320 mg/d in div. doses
Calcium-Channel Blockers			
bepridil hydrochloride	Vascor	PO	Start with 200 mg once/d, may be adjusted q7d (max: 400 mg/d)
diltiazem	Cardizem	PO	30 mg qid, may increase q1–2d as required (usual

(continued)

nicardipine hydrochloride	Cardene	PO, IV	range: 180–360 mg/d in div. doses) PO: 20–40 mg tid or 30–60 mg SR bid; IV: Initiation of therapy in a drug-free patient: 5 mg/h initially, increase dose by 2.5 mg/h q15min (or faster) (max: 15 mg/h)
nifedipine	Adalat, Procardia	PO	10–20 mg tid up to 180 mg/d
nisoldipine	Sular, Nisocor	PO	10–20 mg/d in 2 div. doses (max: 40 mg/d), may need to reduce dose in patients w/liver disease (cirrhosis, chronic hepatitis)
verapamil hydrochloride	Calan, Verelan PM	PO	80 mg q6–8h, may increase up to 320–480 mg/d in div. doses

DRUGS TO TREAT HYPERTENSION

Hypertension is defined as an abnormal increase in arterial blood pressure. Approximately 90 percent of patients have essential hypertension that is of an unknown cause. Untreated hypertension may lead to:

- Heart attack
- Stroke
- Kidney damage
- Blindness

Many classes of drugs are used to treat hypertension, including:

- Diuretics
- Calcium channel blockers
- Beta-blockers
- Alpha-blockers
- Angiotensin converting enzyme inhibitors (ACE inhibitors)

Remember...

Some hypertension drugs have advantages in certain types of patients.

Three types of diuretics are used to treat hypertension. Table 18–16 shows a list of diuretics.

TABLE 18–16 Diuretics

Generic Name	Trade Name	Route of Administration	Average Adult Dosage
Thiazide Diuretics			
chlorothiazide	Diachlor, SK-Chlorothiazide	PO, IV	PO: 250 mg–1 g/d in 1–2 div. doses; IV: 250 mg–1 g/d in 1–2 div. doses
chlorthalidone	Hygroton, Hylidone	PO	12.5–25 mg/d, may be increased to 100 mg/d if needed
hydrochlorothiazide	HydroDIURIL	PO	12.5–200 mg/d in 1–3 div. doses
indapamide	Lozol	PO	2.5 mg once/d, may increase to 5 mg/d if needed
metolazone	Mykrox	PO	0.5–1 mg/d

(continued)

Loop Diuretics

bumetanide	Bumex	PO, IM, IV	PO: 0.5–2 mg once/d, may repeat at 4–5 h intervals if needed (max: 10 mg/d); IV/IM: 0.5–1 mg over 1–2 min, repeated q2–3 h prn (max: 10 mg/d)
ethacrynic acid	Edecrin	PO, IV	PO: 50–100 mg 1–2 times/d, may increase by 25–50 mg prn up to 400 mg/d; IV: 0.5–1 mg/kg or 50 mg up to 100 mg, may repeat prn
furosemide	Lasix	PO, IM, IV	20–80 mg in 1 or more div. doses up to 600 mg/d prn; IM/IV: 20–40 mg in 1 or more div. doses up to 600 mg/d

(continued)

torsemide	Demadex	PO, IV	10–20 mg once/d, may increase up to 200 mg/d prn
Potassium-Sparing Diuretics			
spironolactone	Aldactone	PO	25–200 mg/d in div. doses, continued for at least 5 d (dose adjusted to optimal response; if no response, a thiazide or loop diuretic may be added)
triamterene	Dyrenium	PO	100 mg bid (max: 300 mg/d), may be able to decrease to 100 mg/d or qod
Combination Agents			
amiloride/HCTZ	Moduretic	PO	5 mg/d, may increase up to 20 mg/d in 1–2 div. doses
bisoprolol/HCTZ	Zebeta	PO	2.5–5 mg once/d, may increase to 20 mg/d prn

(continued)

lisinopril/HCTZ	Zestoretic	PO	10 mg once/d, may increase up to 20–40 mg 1–2 times/d (max: 80 mg/d)
losartan/HCTZ	Hyzaar	PO	25–50 mg in 1–2 div. doses (max: 100 mg/d); start w/25 mg/d if volume depleted
spironolactone/HCTZ	Aldactazide	PO	25–200 mg/d in div. doses, continued for at least 5d (dose adjusted to optimal response; if no response, a thiazide or loop diuretic may be added)
triamterene/HCTZ	Dyazide, Maxzide	PO	100 mg bid (max: 300 mg/d), may be able to decrease to 100 mg/d or qod
valsartan/HCTZ	Diovan HCT	PO	80 mg qd (max: 320 mg qd)

(continued)

Calcium Channel Blockers

Dihydropyridines

amlodipine	Norvasc	PO	5–10 mg once/d
felodipine	Plendil	PO	5–10 mg once/d (max: 20 mg/d)
isradipine	DynaCirc	PO	1.25–10 mg bid (max: 20 mg/d)
nicardipine hydrochloride	Cardene, Cardene SR	PO, IV	PO: 20–40 mg tid or 30–60 mg bid; IV: Initiation in a drug-free patient— 5 mg/h initially, increase dose by 2.5 mg/h q15min (or faster) (max: 15 mg/h)
nifedipine	Procardia, Procardia XL, Adalat CC	PO	10–20 mg tid up to 180 mg/d

(continued)

nimodipine	Nimotop	PO	60 mg q4h for 21 d, start therapy within 96 h or subarachnoid hemorrhage
nisoldipine	Sular, Nisocor	PO	10–20 mg/d in 2 div. doses (max: 40 mg/d), may need to reduce dose in patients w/liver disease
Nondihydropyridines			
diltiazem	Cardizem, Dilacor XR, Tiazac	PO, IV	PO: 30 mg qid, may increase q1–2d prn (usual range: 180–360 mg/d in div. doses); IV: 0.25 mg/kg IV bolus over 2 min, if inadequate response, may repeat in 15 min w/ 0.35 mg/kg, followed by a continuous infusion of 5–10 mg/h (max: 15 mg/h for 24 h)

(continued)

| verapamil hydrochloride | Calan, Calan SR, Verelan | PO, IV | PO: 40–80 mg tid or 90–240 mg sustained release 1–2 times/d up to 480 mg/d; IV: 5–10 mg IV direct, may repeat in 15–30 min prn |

Other antihypertensive agents are listed in Table 18–17.

TABLE 18–17 Beta-Blockers, ACE Inhibitors, and ARBs

Generic Name	Trade Name	Route of Administration	Average Adult Dosage
Beta-Blockers			
acebutolol hydrochloride	Sectral	PO	400–800 mg/d in 1–2 div. doses (max: 1200 mg/d)

(continued)

atenolol	Tenormin	PO, IV	PO: 25–50 mg/d, may increase to 100 mg/d; IV: 5 mg of 5 min × 2 doses, then switch to PO
bisoprolol fumarate	Zebeta	PO	2.5–5 mg once/d, may increase to 20 mg/d prn
carteolol hydrochloride	Cartrol	PO	2.5 mg once/d, may increase to 5–10 mg prn (max: 10 mg/d)
carvedilol	Coreg	PO	Start w/3.125 mg bid × 2wks, may double dose q2wks as tolerated up to 25 mg bid if less than 85 kg or 50 mg bid if more than 85 kg
labetalol hydrochloride	Normodyne, Trandate	PO, IV	PO: 100 mg bid, may gradually increase to 200–400 mg bid (max: 1200–2400 mg/d); IV: 20 mg slowly over 2 min, w/40–80 mg q10min prn up to 300 mg total or

(continued)

metoprolol tartrate	Lopressor, Toprol XL	PO, IV	2 mg/min continuous infusion (max: 300 mg total dose) PO: 50–100 mg/d in 2 div. doses, may increase weekly up to 100–400 mg/d; IV: 5 mg q2min for 3 doses, followed by PO therapy
nadolol	Corgard	PO	40 mg once/d, may increase up to 240–320 mg/d in 1–2 div. doses
pindolol	Visken	PO	5 mg bid, may increase by 10 mg/d q2–3wks prn (max: 60 mg/d in 2–3 div. doses)
propranolol hydrochloride	Inderal, Inderal LA	PO, IV	40 mg bid, usually need 160–480 mg/d in div. doses
sotalol	Betapace	PO	Initial dose of 80 mg bid or 160 mg qd taken prior to meals, may

(continued)

			increase q3–4d in 40–160 mg increments (Most patients respond to 240–320 mg/d in 2–3 div. doses. Doses more than 640 mg/d have not been studied.)
timolol maleate	Betimol, Blocadren	PO	10 mg bid, may increase to 60 mg/d in 2 div. doses

ANTIARRHYTHMICS

Arrhythmias are deviations from the normal pattern of the heartbeat. They may occur because of improper impulse generation, conduction, or both. Common arrhythmias originating in the upper and lower chambers of the heart include:

- Atrial fibrillation
- Atrial flutter
- Premature ventricular contractions
- Ventricular tachycardia
- Ventricular fibrillation

Antiarrhythmic drugs are classified according to their effects on the conduction of impulses through the heart and their mechanism of action. Table 18–18 shows classifications of antiarrhythmic drugs.

TABLE 18–18 Classifications of Antiarrhythmic Drugs

Generic Name	Trade Name	Route of Administration	Average Adult Dosage
Class I			
disopyramide phosphate	Napamide, Norpace	PO	Less than 50 kg, 100 mg q6h or 200 mg sustained release q12h; more than 50 kg, 100–200 mg q6h or 300 mg sustained release capsule q12h
flecainide	Tambocor	PO	100 mg q12h, may increase by 50 mg bid q4d (max: 400 mg/d)
lidocaine hydrochloride	Anestacon, Xylocaine	IM, IV, SC	IM/SC: 200–300 mg, may repeat once after 60–90 min; IV: 50–100 mg bolus at a rate of

(continued)

			20–50 mg/min, may repeat in 5 min, then start infusion of 1–4 mg/min immed. after 1st bolus
mexiletine	Mexitil	PO	200–300 mg q8h (max: 1200 mg/d)
procainamide hydrochloride	Procan, Pronestyl	PO, IM, IV	PO: 1 g followed by 250–500 mg q3h or 500 mg–1 g q6h sust. release; IM: 0.5–1 g q4–6h until able to take PO; IV: 100 mg q5min at a rate of 25–50 mg/min until arrhythmia is controlled or 1 g given, then 2–6 mg/min
quinidine polygalacturonate	Cardioquin	PO	275–825 mg q3–4h for 4 or more doses until arrhythmia terminates, then 137.5–275 mg bid–tid
tocainide hydrochloride	Tonocard	PO	1.2–1.8 g/d in 3 div. doses, may increase up to 2.4 g/d

(continued)

Class II (β-adrenergic blockers)

acebutolol hydrochloride	Sectral	PO	200 mg bid increased to 600–1200 mg/d
esmolol hydrochloride	Brevibloc	IV	500 mcg/kg load. Dose followed by 50 mcg/kg/min, may increase dose q5–10min prn (max: 200 mcg/kg/min)
propranolol hydrochloride	Inderal, InnoPran XL	PO, IV	PO: 10–30 mg tid–qid, IV: 0.5–3 mg q4h prn

Class III (drugs that interfere with potassium outflow)

amiodarone hydrochloride	Amio-Aqueous, Cordarone	PO, IV	PO(loading): 800–1600 mg/d in 1–2 doses for 1–3 w; PO(maint.): 400–600 mg/d in 1–2 doses; IV (loading): 150 mg over 10 min followed by 360 mg over next 6 h; IV (maint.):

(continued)

			540 mg over 18 h (0.5 mg/min), may continue at 0.5 mg/min
bretylium tosylate	Bretylol	IM, IV	IM: 5–10 mg/kg, may repeat in 1–2 h if arrhythmia persists, then 5–10 mg/kg q6–8h for maint.; IV: 5 mg/kg rapid injection, may increase to 10 mg/kg and repeat q15–30 min (max: 30 mg/kg/d); may also give by cont. infusion at 1–2 mg/min
Class IV (calcium channel blockers)			
diltiazem	Cardizem, Cartia XT	IV	0.25 mg/kg bolus over 2 min, if inadequate response, may repeat in 15 min w/0.35 mg/kg, followed by a continuous infusion of 5–10 mg/h (max: 15 mg/h for 24 h)

(continued)

| verapamil hydrochloride | Calan, Isoptin | PO, IV | PO: 240–480 mg/d in div. doses; IV: 5–10 mg direct, may repeat in 15–30 min prn |

Other Drugs

| atropine sulfate | Atropisol, Isopto Atropine | IM, IV | IM/IV: 0.5–1 mg q1–2h prn (max: 2 mg) |
| digoxin | Lanoxicaps, Lanoxin | PO, IV | Digitalizing dose-PO: 10–15 mcg/kg (1 mg) in div. doses over 24–48 h; Dig.dose-IV: 10–15 mcg/kg (1 mg) in div. doses over 24 h. Maint dose (PO/IV): 0.1–0.375 mg/d |

HEART FAILURE AND DRUG THERAPY

Heart failure is the inability of the heart muscle to contract with enough force to properly circulate blood. The most common form of heart failure is often referred to as "congestive heart failure." Heart failure may be treated with a variety of drugs and methods, including:

- Cardiac glycosides
- Diuretics
- ACE inhibitors

- Beta-blockers
- Fluid restriction
- Low-sodium diet

Remember...

The role of cardiac glycosides is not well defined, but they have been shown to increase the force of heart muscle contraction in some patients.

Two currently available cardiac glycosides are:

- Digoxin (Lanoxin®)
- Digitoxin

Remember...

Digoxin has a narrow therapeutic index and may have serious toxicities.

ANTIHYPERLIPIDEMIC DRUGS

Diseases associated with plasma lipids can manifest as an elevation in triglyceride levels (**hyperlipidemia**) or as an elevation in the cholesterol level. Medications are not the first line of treatment for hyperlipidemia. Antihyperlipidemic drugs are used only if diet modification and exercise programs fail to lower low-density lipoprotein (LDL), or "bad cholesterol" levels, to normal. Table 18–19 shows a list of lipid-lowering drugs.

TABLE 18–19 Lipid-Lowering Drugs

Generic Name	Trade Name	Route of Administration	Average Adult Dosage
Bile Acid Sequestrants			
cholestyramine resin	LoCHOLEST, Prevalite, Questran	PO	4–8 g bid–qid a.c. and h.s. (less than or equal to 32 g/d)

(continued)

colesevelam hydrochloride	Welchol	PO	3 tablets bid w/meals or 6 tablets qd w/a meal, may be increased to 7 tablets/d
colestipol hydrochloride	Colestid	PO	15–30 g/d in 2–4 doses a.c. and h.s. or 1–2 tabs 1–2 times/d
Fibric Acid Derivatives			
clofibrate	Atromid-S	PO	2 g/d in 2–4 div. doses
fenofibrate	Lofibra, Luxacor, Tricor	PO	54 mg qd (max: 160 mg/d)
gemfibrozil	Lopid	PO	600 mg bid 30 min before a.m. and p.m. meal, may increase up to 1500 mg/d
Niacin (Nicotinic Acid)			
Immediate release	Niacor	Nasal spray	Not in PDR

(continued)

Sustained release	Niaspan, Slo-Niacin	Transdermal patch	25–100 mg 2–5 times/d
Statins			
atorvastatin calcium	Lipitor	PO	Start w/10–40 mg qd, may increase up to 80 mg/d
fluvastatin	Lescol	PO	20 mg h.s., may increase up to 80 mg/d in 1–2 doses
lovastatin	Altoprev, Mevacor, Mevinolin	PO	20–40 mg 1–2 times/d
pravastatin	Pravachol	PO	10–80 mg qd
simvastatin	Zocor	PO	5–40 mg qd (max: 80 mg qd). Patients taking danazol or cyclosporine should not exceed 10 mg qd.

ANTICOAGULANT DRUGS

Clot formation is vital to prevent bleeding from cuts and other injuries. Without clotting, it is possible to bleed to death. Sometimes, however, clot formation is not desired. Anticoagulants are agents that prevent formation of blood clots (thrombi). Table 18–20 shows the most commonly used anticoagulants.

TABLE 18–20 Commonly Used Anticoagulants

Generic Name	Trade Name	Route of Administration	Average Adult Dosage
dicumarol	Bishydroxycoumarin	PO	200–300 mg on day 1, then 25–200 mg/d based on PT time
heparin sodium	Hepalean, Hep-Lock	IV, SC	IV: 5000-U bolus dose, then 20,000–40,000 U infused over 24 h, dose adjusted to maintain desired APTT or 5000–10,000 U piggyback q4–6h; SC:

(continued)

Generic	Trade	Route	Dosage
			10,000–20,000 U followed by 8,000–20,000 U q8–12h
lepirudin	Refludan	IV	0.4 mg/kg initial bolus (max: 44 mg) followed by 0.15 mg/kg/h (max: 16.5 mg/h) for 2–10 d, adjust rate to maintain APTT of 1.5–2.5
warfarin sodium	Coumadin Sodium, Panwarfin	PO, IV	10–15 mg/d for 2–5 d, then 2–10 mg once/d w/dose adjusted to maintain a PT 1.2–2 times control or INR of 2–3
Low Molecular-Weight Heparin			
dalteparin sodium	Fragmin	SC	120 IU/kg bid for at least 5 d
enoxaparin	Lovenox	SC	1 mg/kg q12h or 1.5 mg/kg/d; monitor anti-Xa activity to determine appropriate dose
tinzaparin sodium	Innohep	SC	175 anti-Xa IU/kg q.d. × at least 6 d

MUSCULOSKELETAL SYSTEM

Some of the most common disorders in humans at any age are those affecting the musculoskeletal system. Pain or inflammation of the muscles or joints is common.

SKELETAL MUSCLE RELAXANTS

Skeletal muscle relaxants work by blocking somatic motor nerve impulses through depression of specific neurons within the CNS. These drugs are called **neuromuscular blocking agents**. These agents are listed in Table 18–21.

Remember...

Neuromuscular blocking agents prevent muscles from moving. These drugs have no effect on pain or level of consciousness.

TABLE 18–21 Neuromuscular Blocking Agents

Generic Name	Trade Name	Route of Administration	Average Adult Dosage
Short Duration			
succinylcholine chloride	Anectine, Quelicin, Sucostrin	IM, IV	IM: 2.5–4 mg/kg up to 150 mg; IV: 0.3–1.1 mg/kg administered over 10–30 sec, may give add'l doses prn
Intermediate Duration			
atracurium besylate	Tracrium	IV	0.4–0.5 mg/kg initial dose, then 0.08–0.1 mg/kg 20–45 min after the first dose prn; reduce doses if used with general anesthetics
cisatracurium besylate	Nimbex	IV	Intubation: 0.15 or 0.20 mg/kg;

(continued)

			Maint.: 0.03 mg/kg q20min prn or 1–2 mcg/kg/min
Extended Duration			
doxacurium chloride	Nuromax	IV	0.05 mg/kg administered as rapid bolus injection over 5–10 s. Use lower doses in older adults or patients w/renal or hepatic dysfunction.
mivacurium chloride	Mivacron	IV	(Loading): 0.15 mg/kg given over 5–15 sec (over 60 sec in patients w/cardiovascular disease); Maint.: 0.1 mg/kg generally q15min
pancuronium bromide	Pavulon	IV	0.04–0.1 mg/kg initial dose, may give add'l doses of 0.01 mg/kg at 30–60 min intervals

(continued)

| pipecuronium bromide | Arduan | IV | 85–100 mcg/kg, ideal body weight, given as rapid bolus over 5–10 sec or may give over 1 min if desired |
| tubocurarine chloride | Tubocurarine Chloride | IV | 6–9 mg followed by 3–4.5 mg in 3–5 min prn |

Another group of skeletal muscle relaxants is used orally for painful muscle conditions. These agents are called **centrally acting skeletal muscle relaxants**. Drugs in this group are listed in Table 18–22.

TABLE 18–22 Centrally Acting Skeletal Muscle Relaxants

Generic Name	Trade Name	Route of Administration	Average Adult Dosage
baclofen	Kemstro, Lioresal	PO, Intrathecal	PO: 5 mg tid, may increase by 5 mg/dose q3d prn (max: 80 mg/d); *(continued)*

carisoprodol	Rela, Soma	PO	350 mg tid
chlorzoxazone	Paraflex	PO	250–500 mg tid-qid (max: 3 g/d)
cyclobenzaprine hydrochloride	Cycloflex, Flexeril	PO	5–10 mg tid (max: 60 mg/d)
diazepam	Valium, Valrelease	PO, IM, IV	PO: 2–10 mg bid–qid or 15–30 mg/d sustained release; IM/IV: 2–10 mg, repeat if needed in 3–4 h
methocarbamol	Marbaxin, Robaxin	PO, IM, IV	PO: 1.5 g qid for 2–3 d, then 4–4.5 g/d in 3–6 div. doses; IM: 0.5–1 g q8h; IV: 1–3 g/d in div. doses (max: rate of 300 mg/min)
orphenadrine citrate	Banflex, Norflex	PO, IM, IV	PO: 100 mg bid; IM/IV: 60 mg, may repeat in 12 h prn

Intrathecal: Prior to infusion pump implantation, initiate trial dose of 50 mcg/mL bolus administered by barbotage up to 1 min.

ANALGESICS, ANTIPYRETICS, AND ANTI-INFLAMMATORY DRUGS

Some pain is relieved with opioid analgesics and other pain with nonopioid analgesics. Many nonopioid analgesics affect pain, fever, and inflammation, depending on their properties (see Tables 18–23, 18–24, and 18–25).

TABLE 18–23 Anti-Inflammatory and Analgesic Agent Salicylates

Generic Name	Trade Name	Route of Administration	Average Adult Dosage
aspirin (acetylsalicylic acid)	Alka-Seltzer, Bayer, Ecotrin	PO, Rectal	350–650 mg q4h (max: 4 g/d)
choline magnesium trisalicylate	Trilisate	PO	2–3 g/d in 2 div. doses
choline salicylate	Arthropan	PO	435–870 mg (2.5–5 mL) q4h
magnesium salicylate	Doan's Pills, Magan, Mobidin	PO	650 mg tid-qid

(continued)

| salsalate | Artha-G, Disalcid, Salsitab | PO | 325–3000 mg/d in div. doses (max: 4 g/d) |

TABLE 18–24 Nonsalicylate Anti-Inflammatory and Analgesic Agents (NSAIDs)

Generic Name	Trade Name	Route of Administration	Average Adult Dosage
diclofenac	Cataflam, Solaraze, Voltaren	PO, Ophthalmic, Topical	PO: 150–200 mg/d in 3–4 div. doses; Ophthalmic: 1 drop of 0.1% solution in affected eye qid beginning 24 h after surgery and continuing for 2 w; Topical: Apply to affected area bid for 60–90 d
diflunisal	Dolobid	PO	1000 mg followed by 500 mg q8–12h
etodolac	Lodine, Lodine XL	PO	200–400 mg q6–8h prn

(continued)

fenoprofen calcium	Nalfon	PO	300–600 mg tid–qid (max: 3200 mg/d)
flurbiprofen sodium	Ansaid, Ocufen	PO, Topical	PO: 200–300 mg/d in 2–4 div. doses (max: 300 mg/d); Topical: 1 drop in eye approx q30min beginning 2 h before surgery for a total of 4 drops per affected eye
ibuprofen	Advil, Motrin, Rufen	PO	400–800 mg tid–qid (max: 3200 mg/d)
indomethacin	Indameth, Indocin, Indocin SR	PO, IV, Rectal	PO: 25–50 mg bid–tid (max: 200 mg/d) or 75 mg sustained release 1–2 times/d; IV: less than 48 h, 0.2 mg/kg followed by 2 doses of 0.1 mg/kg q12–24h; 2–7 d, 0.2 mg/kg followed by 2 doses of 0.2 mg/kg q12–24h; less than 7 days, 0.2 mg/kg

(continued)

		followed by 2 doses of 0.25 mg/kg q12–24 h; Rectal: 50 mg tid until pain is tolerable, then rapidly taper
ketoprofen	Actron, Orudis, Oruvail	PO	75 mg tid or 50 mg qid (max: 300 mg/d) or 200 mg sustained release qd
meclofenamate sodium	Meclofen, Meclomen	PO	200–400 mg/d in 3–4 div. doses (max: 400 mg/d)
meloxicam	Mobic	PO	7.5–15 mg once/d
nabumetone	Relafen	PO	1000 mg/d as a single dose, may increase (max: of 2000 mg/d in 1–2 div. doses)
naproxen	EC-Naprosyn, Naprelan, Naprosyn	PO	250–500 mg bid (max: 1000 mg/d)
naproxen sodium	Aleve, Anaprox, Anaprox DS	PO	250–500 mg bid (max: 1100 mg/d)

(continued)

			600–1200 mg qd (max: 1800 mg/d or 25 mg/kg, whichever is lower)
oxaprozin		Daypro	PO
piroxicam		Feldene	PO	10–20 mg 1–2 times/d
sulindac		Clinoril	PO	150–200 mg bid (max: 400 mg/d)
tolmetin sodium		Tolectin, Tolectin DS	PO	400 mg tid (max: 2 g/d)

TABLE 18–25 Second-Line Agents for Rheumatoid Arthritis

Generic Name	Trade Name	Route of Administration	Average Adult Dosage
auranofin	Ridaura	PO	6 mg/d in 1–2 div. doses, may increase to 6–9 mg/d in 3 div. doses after 6 mo. (max: 9 mg/d)
gold sodium thiomalate	Myochrysine	IM	10 mg wk 1, 25 mg wk 2, then 25–50 mg/wk to a cumulative dose

(continued)

			of 1 g (If improvement occurs, continue at 25–50 mg q2w for 2–20 w, then q3–4w indefinitely or until adverse effects occur.)
methotrexate	Amethopterin, Mexate, Rheumatrex	PO	PO: 2.5–5 mg q12h for 3 doses each wk or 7.5 mg once/wk
penicillamine	Cuprimine, Depen	PO	125–250 mg/d; may increase at 1–3 mo. Intervals up to 1–1.5 g/d
sulfasalazine	Azulfidine	PO	1–2 g/d in 4 div. doses, may increase up to 8 g/d prn

IMMUNE SYSTEM

The immune system is the organized collection of mechanisms the body uses to protect itself from invading microorganisms. The immune system includes white blood cells, phagocytic cells in the liver and other organs, and the immunoglobulins. Pathogenic microorganisms produce infections of different organs or systems of the body. Invading microorganisms include:

- Viruses
- Fungi
- Parasites
- Bacteria
- Protozoa

This section emphasizes drugs used to treat bacteria, along with some antivirals and antifungals.

CHAIN OF INFECTION

The chain of infection describes the elements of an infectious process. This process must include several essential elements or "links in the chain" for the transmission of microorganisms to occur. There are six essential links, which include:

1. Infectious agent
2. Reservoir or source
3. Portal of exit from reservoir or source
4. Mode of transmission
5. Portal of entry to host
6. Susceptible host

Antibacterial agents are classified in two groups: bactericidal and bacteriostatic. Table 18–26 shows bactericidal versus bacteriostatic antibacterial agents.

TABLE 18-26 Bactericidal versus Bacteriostatic Antibacterial Agents

Bactericidal Agents	Bacteriostatic Agents
Aminoglycosides	Chloramphenicol
Bacitracin	Clindamycin
Beta-lactam antibiotics	Ethambutol
Isoniazid	Macrolides
Metronidazole	Nitrofurantoin
Polymyxins	Novobiocin
Pyrazinamide	Oxazolidinones
Quinolones	Sulfonamides
Rifampin	Tetracyclines
Vancomycin	Trimethoprim

BETA-LACTAM ANTIBIOTICS

Beta-lactam antibiotics are broad-spectrum and have relatively few adverse effects. Beta-lactam antibiotics include:

- Penicillins
- Cephalosporins
- Carbapenems
- Monobactams

PENICILLINS

Penicillins were one of the first antibiotics developed. They are classified in three groups:

1. Natural penicillins
2. Antistaphylococcal penicillins (Penicillinase-resistant)
3. Extended-spectrum penicillins (Semisynthetic)

Table 18–27 shows common penicillins.

Remember...

Penicillin allergies can be fatal. All patients should be carefully questioned about their allergy histories before they are administered any drug of this class.

TABLE 18-27 Common Penicillins

Generic Name	Trade Name	Route of Administration	Average Adult Dosage
Natural Penicillins			
penicillin G potassium	Pentids, Pfizerpen	PO, IM, IV	PO: 1.6–3.2 million U div. q6h; IM/IV: 1.2–24 million U div. q4h
penicillin G benzathine	Bicillin, Permapen	IM	1,200,000 U once/d
penicillin G procaine	Crysticillin A.S., Wycillin	IM	600,000–1,200,000 U once/d
penicillin V potassium	Beepen VK, Ledercillin VK	PO	125–500 mg q6h
Penicillinase-Resistant Penicillins			
cloxacillin sodium	Cloxapen, Cloxilean	PO	250–500 mg q6h
dicloxacillin sodium	Dycill, Dynapen	PO	250–500 mg q6h

(continued)

nafcillin sodium	Nafcil, Unipen	PO, IM, IV	PO: 250–1000 mg q4–6h; IM/IV: 500 mg–2g q4–6h up to 12 g/d
oxacillin sodium	Bactocill, Prostaphlin	PO, IM, IV	PO: 250–1000 mg q4–6h; IM/IV: 500 mg–2 g q4–6h up to 12 g/d
Semisynthetic Penicillins			
amoxillin	Amoxil, Trimox	PO	250–500 mg q8h
amoxicillin/clavulanate potassium	Augmentin, Augmentin XR	PO	250 or 500 mg tablet (each w/125 mg clavulanic acid) q8–12h; sustained released tabs: 2 tabs (2000 mg amoxicillin/ 125 mg clavulanate) q12h × 7–10 d
ampicillin	Ampicin, Omnipen	PO, IM, IV	PO: 250–500 mg q6h; IM/IV: 250 mg–2 g q6h
bacampicillin hydrochloride	Spectrobid	PO	400–800 mg q12h

CEPHALOSPORINS

Cephalosporins are semisynthetic antibiotics structurally and pharmacologically related to penicillins. The cephalosporins are classified into four different "generations" (see Table 18-28).

TABLE 18-28 Classifications of Cephalosporins

Generic Name	Trade Name	Route of Administration	Average Adult Dosage
First Generation			
cefadroxil	Duricef, Ultracef	PO	1–2 g/d in 1–2 div. doses
cefazolin sodium	Ancef, Kefzol	IM, IV	250 mg–2 g q8h, up to 2 g q4h (max: 12 g/d)
cephalexin	Cefanex, Keflex	PO	250–500 mg q6h

(continued)

cephradine	Anspor, Velosef	PO, IM, IV	PO: 250–500 mg q6h or 500 mg–1 g q12h up to 4 g/d; IM/IV: 2–4 g/d in 4 div. doses (max: 8 g/d)
Second Generation			
cefaclor	Ceclor, Ceclor CD	PO	250–500 mg q8h (Ceclor), or 250–500 mg/q12h (Ceclor CD)
cefamandole nafate	Mandol	IM, IV	IM/IV: 500 mg–1 g q4–8h, up to 2 g q4h
cefonicid sodium	Monocid	IM, IV	IM/IV: 1 g q24h, up to 2 g/24h
cefotetan disodium	Cefotan	IM, IV	IM/IV: 1–2 g q12h
cefoxitin sodium	Mefoxin	IM, IV	IM/IV: 1–2 g q6–8h, up to 12 g/d
cefuroxime sodium	Kefurox, Zinacef	PO, IM, IV	PO: 250–500 mg q12h; IM/IV: 750 mg–1.5 g q6–8h
Third Generation			
cefdinir	Omnicef	PO	300 mg q12h × 10 d

(continued)

cefixime	Suprax	PO	400 mg/d in 1–2 div. doses
cefoperazone sodium	Cefobid	IM, IV	IM/IV: 1–2 g q12h; 16 g/d in 2–4 div. doses
cefotaxime sodium	Claforan	IM, IV	IM/IV: 1–2 g q8–12h, up to 2 g q4h (max: 12 g/d)
cefpodoxime	Vantin	PO	200 mg q12h for 10 d
cefprozil	Cefzil	PO	250–500 mg q12–24h for 10–14 d
ceftazidime	Fortaz, Tazicef	IM, IV	IM/IV: 1–2 g q8–12h, up to 2 g q6 h
ceftibuten	Cedax	PO	400 mg once/d for 10 d
ceftizoxime sodium	Cefizox	IM, IV	IM/IV: 1–2 g q8–12h, up to 2 g q4h
ceftriaxone sodium	Rocephin	IM, IV	IM/IV: 1–2 g q12–24h (max: 4 g/d)
Fourth Generation			
cefepime hydrochloride	Maxipime	IM, IV	IM/IV: 0.5–1 g q12 h × 7–10 d

MACROLIDES

Macrolides are especially useful against respiratory infections. Table 18–29 shows common macrolides.

Remember...

Patients who are allergic to penicillins can usually take any of the macrolides.

TABLE 18–29 Common Macrolides

Generic Name	Trade Name	Route of Administration	Average Adult Dosage
azithromycin	Zithromax	PO, IV	PO: 500 mg day 1, then 250 mg q24h for 4 d; IV: 500 mg qd for at least 2 d, administer 1 mg/mL over 3 h or 2 mg/mL over 1 h

(continued)

clarithromycin	Biaxin Filmtabs, Biaxin XL	PO	250–500 mg bid for 10–14 d (For the XL formulation, use 500 mg qd for 10–14 d.)
dirithromycin	Dynabac	PO	500 mg once/d
erythromycin	Erythrocin, Ilotycin	PO	250–500 mg q6h; 333 mg q8h
erythromycin estolate	Ilosone	PO	250–500 mg q6h; 333 mg q8h
erythromycin gluceptate	Ilotycin Gluceptate	IV	250 mg–1 g q6h up to 4 g/d according to severity of infection
erythromycin ethylsuccinate	E.E.S., EryPed	PO	400 mg q6h up to 4 g/d according to severity of infection
troleandomycin	Tao	PO	250–500 mg q6h

SULFONAMIDES

Sulfonamides were the first drugs to successfully prevent and cure human bacterial infections. The major sulfonamides are generally classified as:

- Short-acting
- Intermediate-acting
- Long-acting

See Table 18–30 for a classification of sulfonamides.

Remember...

Hematuria and crystalluria are two of the major adverse effects of sulfonamide agents. They should be used with caution in patients with kidney impairment.

Remember...

The patient should be advised to take in adequate fluids to prevent or minimize the risks of renal damage while taking sulfonamides.

TABLE 18–30 Classifications of Sulfonamides

Generic Name	Trade Name	Route of Administration	Average Adult Dosage
Short-Acting Sulfonamides			
sulfisoxazole	Gantrisin	PO, Vaginal	PO: 2–4 g initially, followed by 4–8 g/d in 4–6 div. doses; Vaginal: 1 applicator full 1–2 times/d
Intermediate-Acting Sulfonamides			
sulfadiazine	Microsulfon	PO	Loading dose: 2–4 g; Maint. dose: 2–4 g/d in 4–6 div. doses
sulfamethoxazole	Sulfamethoxazole	PO	Loading dose: 2 g; Maint. dose: 1 g q8–12h

(continued)

Long-Acting Sulfonamides			
sulfasalazine	Azulfidine	PO	1–2 g/d in 4 div. doses, may increase up to 8 g/d prn
Combination Sulfonamides			
trimethoprim/sulfamethoxazole	Bactrim, Co-Trimoxazole, Septra	PO, IV	PO: 160 mg TMP/800 mg SMZ (1 double-strength tablet) q12h; IV: 8–10 mg/kg/d TMP divided q6–12h infused over 60–90 min
sulfadiazine/sulfamerazine/sulfamethazine	Triple Sulfa, Sultrin	PO	Combination tablet (sulfadiazine 167 mg, sulfamerazine 167 mg, sulfamethazine 167 mg)/d

TETRACYCLINES

Tetracyclines are broad-spectrum agents that are effective against certain bacterial strains that are resistant to other antibiotics. The major tetracyclines are shown in Table 18–31.

Remember...

Tetracyclines are able to combine with iron, calcium, aluminum, and magnesium. Therefore, they should not be given with iron tablets, antacids, or dairy products.

Remember...

Tetracyclines should not be used in children younger than eight years of age unless other appropriate drugs are ineffective or contraindicated.

TABLE 18-31 Classifications of Tetracyclines

Generic Name	Trade Name	Route of Administration	Average Adult Dosage
Short-Acting			
oxytetracycline	Terramycin	PO, IM, IV	PO: 250–500 mg q6–12h; IM: 100 mg q8–12h; IV: 250–500 mg q12h (max: 500 mg q6h)
tetracycline hydrochloride	Achromycin, Sumycin	PO, IM, Topical	PO: 250–500 mg bid–qid (1–2 g/d);

(continued)

Intermediate-Acting		
demeclocycline hydrochloride	Declomycin	PO	IM: 250 mg once/d or 300 mg/d in 2–3 div. doses; Topical: Apply to cleansed areas twice/d
			150 mg q6h or 300 mg q12h (max: 2.4 g/d)
Long-Acting		
doxycycline	Adoxa, Vibramycin	PO, IV	PO/IV: 100 mg q12h on day 1, then 100 mg/d as single dose (max: 100 mg q12h)
hyclateminocycline hydrochloride	Dynacin, Minocin	PO, IV	PO/IV: 200 mg followed by 100 mg q12h

AMINOGLYCOSIDES

Aminoglycosides are used primarily for infections caused by gram-negative enterobacteria. The toxic potential of these drugs limits their use. Major aminoglycosides are shown in Table 18–32.

Remember...

Aminoglycosides can cause serious adverse effects such as ototoxicity and nephrotoxicity. Neomycin is the most nephrotoxic aminoglycoside, and streptomycin is the least nephrotoxic.

TABLE 18–32 Most Commonly Used Aminoglycosides

Generic Name	Trade Name	Route of Administration	Average Adult Dosage
amikacin sulfate	Amikin	IM, IV	IM/IV: 5–7.5 mg/kg loading dose, then 7.5 mg/kg q12h
gentamicin sulfate	Garamycin, Genoptic	IM, IV, Intrathecal, Ophthalmic, Topical	IM/IV: 1.5–2 mg/kg loading dose, followed by 3–5 mg/kg/d in 2–3 div. doses; Intrathecal: 4–8 mg preservative free qd; Ophthalmic: 1–2 drops of solution in eye q4h up to 2 drops

(continued)

			qh; Topical: Small amount of ointment bid–tid
kanamycin	Kantrex	PO, IM, IV, Inhalation, Intraperitoneal, Irrigation	PO: 1 g qh for 4 doses, then q6h for 36–72 h; IM/IV: 15 mg/kg/d in equally div. doses q8–12h; Inhalation: 250 mg diluted in 3 mL NS administered per nebulizer q6–12h; Intraperitoneal: 500 mg diluted in 20 mL sterile water instilled through wound catheter; Irrigation: 0.25% solution prn
neomycin sulfate	Mycifradin, Neo-Tabs	PO, IM, Topical	PO: 1 g qh × 4 doses, then 1 g q4h × 5 doses; IM: 1.3–2.6 mg/kg q6h; Topical: Apply 1–3 times/d
netilmicin sulfate	Netromycin	IM, IV	IM/IV: 1.3–2.2 mg/kg q8h or 2–3.25 mg/kg q12h
streptomycin sulfate	Streptomycin	IM	15 mg/kg up to 1 g/d as single dose

(continued)

| tobramycin sulfate | Nebcin, Tobrex | IM, IV, Inhalation, Ophthalmic | IM: 3 mg/kg/d divided q8h up to 5 mg/kg/d; IV: 3 mg/kg/d divided q8h up to 5 mg/kg/d infused over 20–60 min; Inhalation: 300 mg inhaled via nebulizer bid × 28 d, may repeat after 28 d drug-free period; Ophthalmic: 1–2 drops in affected eye q1–4h |

FLUOROQUINOLONES

Fluoroquinolones are related to nalidixic acid. These agents may be useful in penicillin-allergic patients. The most commonly used fluoroquinolones are shown in Table 18–33.

TABLE 18–33 Most Commonly Used Fluoroquinolones

Generic Name	Trade Name	Route of Administration	Average Adult Dosage
cinoxacin	Cinobac	PO	1 g/d in 2–4 div. doses
ciprofloxacin hydrochloride	Cipro, Cipro IV	PO, IV	PO: 250 mg q12h × 3 d; IV: 200 mg q12h, infused over 60 min
ciprofloxacin ophthalmic	Ciloxan	Ophthalmic, Ointment	Ophthalmic: 1–2 drops in conjunctival sac q2h while awake for 2 d, then 1–2 drops q4h while awake for the next 5 d; Ointment: $\frac{1}{2}$-inch ribbon into conjunctival sac tid × 2 d, then bid × 5 d
gatifloxacin	Tequin	PO, IV	PO/IV: 400 mg qd × 5 d

(continued)

levofloxacin	Iquix, Levaquin	PO, IV, Ophthalmic	PO: 500 mg q24h × 10 d; IV: 500 mg infused over 60 min q24h × 7–14 d; Ophthalmic: Days 1–2, instill 1–2 drops in affected eye(s) q2h while awake (max: 8 times/d); days 3–7, instill 1–2 drops in affected eye(s) q4h while awake (max: 4 times/d)
moxifloxacin hydrochloride	Avelox, Vigamox	PO, IV, Ophthalmic	PO/IV: 400 mg qd × 5–10 d; Ophthalmic: 1 drop in affected eye(s) tid × 7 d
nalidixic acid	NegGram	PO	Acute therapy: 1 g qid; Chronic therapy: 500 mg qid
nitrofurantoin	Furadantin, Furalan	PO	50–100 mg qid
norfloxacin	Chibroxin, Noroxin	PO, Ophthalmic	PO: 400 mg bid; Ophthalmic: 1–2 drops qid

(continued)

ofloxacin	Floxin, Ocuflox	PO, IV, Ophthalmic, Otic	PO: 200–400 mg q12h × 7–10 d; IV: 400 mg q12h × 7 d; Ophthalmic: Instill 1–2 drops q2–4h for first 2 d, then qid for up to 5 d; Otic: 10 drops (0.5 mL) q12h for 14 d
sparfloxacin	Zagam	PO	400 mg day 1, then 200 mg qd days 2–10

MISCELLANEOUS ANTIBACTERIAL AGENTS

Some antibiotics are classified as miscellaneous antibacterial agents, such as chloramphenicol, clindamycin, metronidazole, and vancomycin.

- **Chloramphenicol:** Because of potential toxicity, bacterial resistance, and the availability of other effective drugs (for example, cephalosporins), chloramphenicol is not used as widely as it once was.

- **Clindamycin:** Clindamycin is effective against many organisms found on the skin and in the mouth. It has marked toxicity.

- **Metronidazole:** Metronidazole is the most effective antibiotic against anaerobic bacteria (bacteria that grow without oxygen). Anaerobic bacteria cause infections primarily in the abdomen and vagina.

Remember...

To prevent a severe drug reaction, patients taking metronidazole must avoid alcohol.

- **Vancomycin:** Vancomycin can destroy most gram-positive organisms. It is also useful for treating infections in patients who are allergic to penicillin.

Remember...

Vancomycin is usually given intravenously. It should be well diluted and given slowly. A reaction, referred to as Red Man Syndrome, may occur if the drug is given too rapidly.

ANTIVIRAL DRUGS

Antivirals are used to treat viral infections; they act by influencing viral replication. The majority of antiviral drugs are active against only one type of virus, either the DNA or the RNA type. DNA viruses include:

- Herpes simplex virus (HSV) 1 and 2
- Varicella-zoster virus (VZV)
- Cytomegalovirus (CMV)
- Influenza A virus

Table 18–34 shows antiviral agents that are currently approved for the treatment of DNA viruses.

TABLE 18–34 Antivirals for the Treatment of DNA Viruses

Generic Name	Trade Name	Route of Administration	Average Adult Dosage
acyclovir, aciclovir sodium	Acycloguanosine, Zovirax	PO, IV, Topical	PO: 200 mg q4h 5 times/d, 400 mg tid for 7–10 d cycle; IV: 5 mg/kg q8h; Topical: Apply q3h 6 times/d for 7 d

(continued)

amantadine hydrochloride	Symmetrel	PO	200 mg once/d or 100 mg q12h
cidofovir	Vistide	IV	5 mg/kg once/wk for 2 wk; also give 2 g probenecid 3 h prior to infusion and 1 g 8 h after infusion (4 g total)
famciclovir	Famvir	PO	500 mg q8h × 7 d, start within 48–72 h of onset of rash
foscarnet	Foscavir	IV	Induction: 60 mg/kg infused over 1 h q8h for 2–3 wk; induction may be repeated if relapse occurs during maint. therapy
ganciclovir	Cytovene	PO, IV	PO: 1000 mg tid or 500 mg 6 times/d q3h while awake; IV: 5 mg/kg over 1 h q12h for 14–21 d (Doses may range from 2.5–5 mg/kg over 1 h q8–12h for 10–35 d.)

(continued)

oseltamivir phosphate	Tamiflu	PO	75 mg bid × 5 d
ribavirin	Rebetol, Virazole	PO, Inhalation	PO: Over 75 kg, 600 mg bid for 24–48 wk; under 75 kg, 400 mg in a.m., 600 mg in p.m. for 24–48 wk; Inhalation: 20 mg via SPAG nebulizer administered over 12–18 h/d for a min. of 3 d (max: 7 d)
rimantadine	Flumadine	PO	100 mg bid, reduce to 100 mg/d in older adults or patients w/liver disease
tenofovir disoproxil fumarate	Viread	PO	300 mg once/d w/meal
valacyclovir hydrochloride	Valtrex	PO	1 g (2 × 500 mg) tid for 7 d, start within 48 h of onset of rash
valganciclovir hydrochloride	Valcyte	PO	900 mg bid w/food × 21 d

(continued)

| zanamivir | Relenza | Inhalation | 2 inhalations (one 5 mg blister per inhalation) bid (approx. 12 h apart) × 5 d |

RNA viruses include:

- Picornavirus (polio)
- Rhabdovirus (rabies)
- Paramyxovirus (mumps and measles)
- Retrovirus (HIV)

Most patients with HIV infection are receiving combination therapy with different antiviral agents. Presently, three classes of antiretroviral agents effective against HIV-1 and HIV-2 have been approved. They include:

1. Nucleoside reverse transcriptase inhibitors (NRTIs)
2. Non-nucleoside reverse transcriptase inhibitors (NNRTIs)
3. Protease inhibitors (PIs)

Table 18–35 shows classifications of HIV antiviral agents.

TABLE 18–35 Classifications of HIV Antiviral Agents

Generic Name	Trade Name	Route of Administration	Average Adult Dosage
NRTIs			
abacavir sulfate	Ziagen	PO	300 mg bid
didanosine (DDI)	Videx, Videx EC	PO	Based on weight, 125–400 mg qd–bid
lamivudine (3TC)	Epivir	PO	150 mg bid
stavudine (d4T)	Zerit	PO	Based on weight, 30–40 mg q12h
zalcitabine (ddC, dideoxycytidine)	Hivid	PO	0.01 mg/kg q8h
zidovudine (azidothymidine, AZT)	Retrovir	PO, IV	PO: 200 mg q4h (1200 mg/d), after 1 mo may reduce to 100 mg q4h

(continued)

			(600 mg/d); IV: 1–2 mg/kg q4h (1200 mg/d)
NNRTIs			
delavirdine mesylate	Rescriptor	PO	400 mg tid
efavirenz	Sustiva	PO	600 mg qd
nevirapine	Viramune	PO	200 mg once/d for first 14 d, then increase to 200 mg bid
PIs			
amprenavir	Agenerase	PO	1200 mg capsules bid
indinavir sulfate	Crixivan	PO	800 mg (2 × 400 mg) q8h 1 h before or 2 h after meal
nelfinavir mesylate	Viracept	PO	750 mg tid or 1250 mg (2 × 625 mg) bid w/food

(continued)

ritonavir	Norvir	PO	600 mg bid 1 h before or 2 h after meal (may take with a light snack)
saquinavir mesylate	Fortovase, Invirase	PO	Fortovase: 1200 mg (6 × 200 mg) tid w/meals; Invirase: 600 mg (3 × 200 mg) tid taken 2 h after a full meal
tenofovir disoproxil fumarate	Viread	PO	

HIGHLY ACTIVE ANTIRETROVIRAL THERAPY (HAART)

Antiviral agents are used either alone, or in combination, for the treatment of HIV infection. HAART has been shown to offer the following effects:

- Reduction of viral load
- Increase of CD4 lymphocytes in persons infected with HIV
- Delaying the onset of AIDS
- Prolonging survival of patients with AIDS

HAART involves the combination of three to four drugs that are effective against HIV. Two distinct categories of drugs are combined:

1. Nucleoside analogs   2. Protease inhibitors

ANTIFUNGALS

Antifungals are often used to treat systemic, local fungal, and topical fungal infections. Antifungal drugs are listed in Table 18–36.

TABLE 18–36 Most Commonly Used Antifungal Agents

Generic Name	Trade Name	Route of Administration	Average Adult Dosage
amphotericin B	Amphocin, Fungizone	PO, IV, Irrigation, Topical	PO (Fungizone): 100 mg swish & swallow qid; IV (Amphocin): 1 mg dissolved in 20 mL of D5W by slow infusion (over 10–30 min); Irrigation (Amphocin & Fungizone): 5–50 mg/ 1000 mL sterile water instilled continuously into the bladder via a

(continued)

			3-way closed drainage catheter system at a rate of 1000 mL/24 h;
butenafine hydrochloride	Mentax	Topical	Topical (Fungizone): Apply to lesions 2–4 times/d for 1–4 wks
			Apply to affected area and surrounding skin bid × 7 d or qd × 4 wks
caspofungin acetate	Cancidas	IV	Loading dose: 70 mg; maint. dose: 50 mg qd
ciclopirox olamine	Loprox, Penlac Nail Lacquer	Topical	Massage cream into affected area and surrounding skin twice/d, a.m. and p.m.
clotrimazole	Lotrimin, Mycelex	PO, Topical, Vaginal	PO: 1 troche 5 times/d q3h for 14 d; Topical: Apply small amount onto affected areas bid a.m. and p.m.; Vaginal: Insert 1 application full or one 100 mg vaginal tablet into vagina

(continued)

			at bedtime for 7 d, or one 500 mg vaginal tablet at bedtime for 1 dose
econazole nitrate	Spectazole	Topical	Apply sufficient amount to affected areas twice/d, a.m. and p.m.
fluconazole	Diflucan	PO, IV	PO/IV: 200 mg day 1, then 100 mg qd × 2 wks
flucytosine	Ancobon, 5-FC	PO	50–150 mg/kg/d divided q6h
griseofulvin micro-size	Fulvicin-U/F; Grisactin	PO	500 mg micro-size or 330–375 mg ultramicrosize daily in single or div. doses
itraconazole	Sporanox	PO, IV	PO: 200 mg once/d (increase to max. 200 mg bid if no apparent improvement)—continue for at least 3 mo; for life-threatening infections, start w/200 mg tid for 3 d, then 200–400 mg/d;

(continued)

ketoconazole	Nizoral, Nizoral A-D	PO, Topical	IV: 200 mg bid infused over 1 h for 4 doses, then 200 mg qd; PO: 200–400 mg once/d; Topical: Apply 1–2 times/d to affected area and surrounding skin
miconazole nitrate	Monistat 3, Monistat 7	Topical, Vaginal	Topical: Apply cream sparingly to affected areas twice/d, and once daily for tinea versicolor, for 2 wk (improvement expected in 2–3 d, tinea pedis is treated for 1 mo to prevent recurrence); Vaginal: Insert suppository or vaginal cream q h.s. times 7 d (100 mg) or 3 d (200 mg)
nystatin	Mycostatin, Nilstat	PO, Vaginal	PO: 500,000–1,000,000 U tid; 1–4 troches 4–5 times/d; suspension 400,000–600,000 U qid; Vaginal: 1–2 tablets daily for 2 wk

(continued)

| terbinafine hydrochloride | Lamisil, Lamisil DermaGel | PO, Topical | PO: 250 mg qd × 6 wk for fingernails or times 12 wk for toenails; Topical: Apply qd or bid to affected and immediately surrounding areas until clinical signs and symptoms are significantly improved (1–7 wk). |
| voriconazole | Vfend | PO, IV | PO (over 40kg), 400 mg q12h day 1, then 200 mg q12h, may increase to 300 mg q12h if inadequate response; (under 40kg), 400 mg q12h day 1, then 100 mg q12h, may increase to 150 mg q12h if inadequate response; IV: 6 mg/kg q12h day 1, then 4 mg/kg q12h, may reduce to 3 mg/kg q12h if not tolerated |

RESPIRATORY SYSTEM

Upper respiratory tract infections are more common than lower respiratory track infections, and may be caused by viruses, bacteria, or fungi. Upper respiratory tract infections can be treated by appropriate antibiotics, as discussed earlier. Lower respiratory tract infections are less common, and the lungs are the primary site of tuberculosis and pneumonia.

ANTITUBERCULAR DRUGS

The primary lesion of tuberculosis is located in the lungs. The patient's resistance to secondary tuberculosis depends on general health and environment. In the United States, certain groups of the population are more prone to acquire active tuberculosis. These people include:

- Patients with AIDS
- Drug abusers
- Homeless shelter residents
- Nursing home residents

Antitubercular drugs are used to treat tuberculosis. Primary antitubercular drugs include:

- Isoniazid
- Rifampin
- Streptomycin
- Ethambutol
- Pyrazinamide

ANTINEOPLASTIC DRUGS

Antineoplastic agents are used to treat cancers. Generally, there are three types of treatments, or combinations of treatments, which include:

1. Surgery   2. Radiation   3. Chemotherapy (drug therapy)

The common types of antineoplastic drugs are shown in Table 18–37.

TABLE 18-37 Common Antineoplastic Agents

Generic Name	Trade Name	Route of Administration	Average Adult Dosage
Antimetabolites			
fluorouracil (5-FU)	Adrucil, Efudex	IV, Topical	IV: 12 mg/kg/d for 4 consecutive days up to 800 mg or until toxicity develops or 12 d therapy, may repeat at 1 mo

(continued)

			intervals; if toxicity occurs, 15 mg/kg once/wk can be given until toxicity subsides; Topical: Apply cream or solution bid for 2–4 wk
mercaptopurine (6-MP)	Purinethol	PO	Loading: 2.5 mg/kg/d, may increase up to 5 mg/kg/d after 4 wk prn; maint.: 1.25–2.5 mg/kg/d
methotrexate	Amethopterin, Mexate	PO, IM, IV	PO/IM/IV: 15–30 mg/d for 5 d, repeat q12wk for 3–5 courses
Hormonal Agents			
Corticosteroids			
dexamethasone	Aeroseb-Dex, Decaderm	PO, IM, IV	PO: 0.25–4 mg bid–qid; IM: 8–16 mg q1–3 wk or 0.8–1.6 mg intralesional q1–3 wk; IV: 10 mg followed by 4 mg q4h, reduce dose after 2–4 d then taper over 5–7 d

(continued)

prednisone	Deltasone, Meticorten	PO	5–60 mg/d in single or div. doses
Gonadotropins			
danazol	Danocrine	PO	100–400 mg in 2 div. doses, start during menstruation or if pregnancy test is negative
fluoxymesterone	Halotestin	PO	10–40 mg/d in div. doses
testolactone	Teslac	PO	250 mg qid
Estrogens			
estramustine phosphate sodium	Emcyt	PO	14 mg/kg/d in 3–4 div. doses
Androgens			
fluoxymesterone	Halotestin	PO	10–40 mg/d in div. doses
Testolactone	Teslac	PO	250 mg qid

(continued)

Antiandrogens

bicalutamide	Casodex	PO	50 mg once/d
flutamide	Eulexin	PO	250 mg (2 caps) q8h
goserelin acetate	Zoladex	SC Implant	3.6 mg once q28h; 10.8 mg depot q12w

Progestins

megestrol acetate	Megace	PO	40 mg qid

Antitumor Antibiotics

bleomycin sulfate	Blenoxane	IM, IV, SC	IM/IV/SC: 10–20 U/m² or 0.25–0.5 U/kg 1–2 times/wk (max: 300–400 U)
daunorubicin hydrochloride	Cerubidine	IV	As a single agent, 30–60 mg/m²/d for 3–5 d q3–4 wk (max: total cumulative dose 500–600 mg/m²)

(continued)

doxorubicin hydrochloride	Adriamycin, Rubex	IV	60–75 mg/m² as single dose at 21 d intervals or 30 mg/m² on each of 3 consecutive days repeated q4wk (max: total cum. dose 500–550 mg/m²)
mitomycin	Mutamycin	IV	20 mg/m²/d as a single dose q6–8wk, add'l doses based on hematologic response
plicamycin	Mithracin, Mithramycin	IV	25–30 mcg/kg once/d for 8–10 d or until toxicity necessitates discontinuing (max: 30 mcg/kg/d for 10 d)

SENSORY SYSTEM

Sensory receptors are specialized cells or cell processes that provide the central nervous system with information about conditions inside or outside the body. General senses are localized in the skin, while the special senses include vision (sight), hearing, taste, and smell.

TOPICAL MEDICATIONS

Topical medications are applied to the surface of the body. The effects of topically administered drugs are usually local. The vast majority of drugs are applied to the:

- Skin
- Eye
- Ear

DRUGS USED FOR SKIN DISEASES

Dermatitis and hypersensitivity reactions are common diseases of the skin. Examples of dermatitis are:

- Poison ivy
- Sunburn
- Psoriasis

A variety of agents are used for skin diseases or conditions. The common types of drugs used for the skin are shown in Table 18–38.

TABLE 18-38 Common Medications Used for the Skin

Generic Name	Trade Name	Route of Administration	Average Adult Dosage
Antibacterial agents			
clindamycin hydrochloride	Cleocin	Topical	Apply to affected areas bid; 1% foam qd application
mupirocin	Bactroban	Topical	Apply to affected area tid, if no response in 3–5 d, reevaluate (usually continue for 1–2 wk)
Antibiotics			
dicloxacillin sodium	Dycill, Dynapen	PO	125–500 mg q6h
tetracycline hydrochloride	Topicycline	Topical	Not used topically for adults Apply to cleansed areas twice daily

(continued)

Antifungal agents

clotrimazole	Lotrimin, Mycelex	PO, Topical	PO: 1 troche (lozenge) 5 times/d q3h for 14 d; Topical: Apply small amount onto affected areas bid a.m. and p.m.
fluconazole	Diflucan	PO, IV	PO/IV: 200 mg day 1, then 100 mg qd × 2 wk
ketoconazole	Nizoal, Nizoral A-D	PO, Topical	PO: 200–400 mg once/d; Topical: Apply 1–2 times/d to affected area and surrounding skin
miconazole nitrate	Monistat-Derm, Micatin	Topical, Vaginal	Topical: Apply cream sparingly to affected areas twice/d, and once/d for tinea versicolor, for 2 wk (improvement expected in 2–3d, tinea pedis is treated in 2–3d to prevent recurrence); Vaginal: Insert suppository or vaginal cream q h.s. × 7 d (100 mg) or 3 d (200 mg)

(continued)

terbinafine hydrochloride	Lamisil, Lamisil DermaGel	PO, Topical	PO: 250 mg qd × 6 wk for fingernails or × 12 wk for toenails; Topical: Apply qd or bid to affected and immediately surrounding areas until clinical signs and symptoms are significantly improved (1–7 wk)
Antiviral agents			
Famciclovir	Famvir	PO	500 mg q8h × 7 d, start within 48–72 h of onset of rash
valacylovir hydrochloride	Valtrex	PO	1 g (2 × 500 mg) t.i.d. for 7 days, start within 48 h of onset of zoster rash
Biologics			
efalizumab	Raptiva	SC	0.7 mg/kg first dose, then 1 mg/kg (max: 200 mg) 1 ×/wk

(continued)

Corticosteroids			
prednisone	Deltasone, Meticorten	PO	5–60 mg/d in single or div. doses
Immunosuppressants			
azathioprine	Azasan, Imuran	PO, IV	PO: 3–5 mg/kg/d initially, may be able to reduce to 1–3 mg/kg/d; IV: 3–5 mg/kg/d initially, may be able to reduce to 1–3 mg/kg/d
methotrexate	Amethopterin, Mexate	PO, IM, IV	PO: 15–30 mg/d for 5 d, repeat q12wk for 3–5 courses; IM/IV: 15–30 mg/d for 5 d, repeat q12wk for 3–5 courses
Retinoids			
tazarotene	Avage, Tazorac	Topical	Apply thin film to affected area once/d in p.m.
tretinoin	Avita, Retin-A	Topical	Apply once/d h.s.

OPHTHALMIC MEDICATIONS

Most of the drugs used in ophthalmology are administered locally. The most common ophthalmic diseases are:

- Conjunctivitis
- Dryness of the eyes
- Glaucoma

The most common types of drugs used for eye disorders are shown in Table 18–39.

Remember...

Ophthalmic preparations must be sterile to prevent eye infections, and should be isotonic to minimize burning.

TABLE 18–39 Commonly Used Medications for Eye Disorders

Generic Name	Trade Name	Route of Administration	Average Adult Dosage
Anti-infective and anti-inflammatory agents			
ciprofloxacin ophthalmic	Ciloxan	Ophthalmic	1–2 drops in conjunctival sac q2h while awake for 2 d, then 1–2 drops q4h while awake for the next 5 d
erythromycin	Ilotycin	Ophthalmic	NOTE: Not used this way in adults
gentamicin sulfate	Garamycin, Genoptic	Ophthalmic	1–2 drops of solution in eye q4h up to 2 drops qh or small amount of ointment bid–tid
tobramycin sulfate	Nebcin, Tobrex	Ophthalmic	1–2 drops in affected eye q1–4h
Antiseptic agents			
benzalkonium chloride	Benza, Zephiran	Ophthalmic	1:10,000–1:2000 solution

(continued)

tetrahydrozoline hydrochloride	Collyrium, Optigene	Ophthalmic	1–2 drops of 0.05% solution in eye bid–tid
Antifungal agents			
natamycin	Natacyn	Ophthalmic	1 drop in conjunctival sac of infected eye q1–2h for 3–4 d; then decrease to 1 drop q6–8h, then gradually decrease to 1 drop q4–7d
Antiviral agents			
idoxuridine (IDU)	Herplex Liquifilm, IDU	Ophthalmic	1 drop instilled in conjunctival sac qh during the day and q2h at night until improvement occurs, then decrease to q2h during the day and q4h at night; use ointment q4h during the day with the last dose at bedtime (5 applications/d)

(continued)

Trifluridine	Viroptic	Ophthalmic	1 drop 1% ophthalmic solution into affected eye q2h during waking hours until healing has occurred (max: 9 drops/d)
vidarabine	Adenine Arabinoside, Vira-A	Ophthalmic	Instill 1 cm ($\frac{1}{2}$ in.) ribbon of ointment into lower conjunctival sac q3h 5 times/d
Corticosteroids			
dexamethasone	Decadron, Maxidex	Ophthalmic	1–2 drops in conjunctival sac up to 4–6 times/d; may instill hourly for severe disease
hydrocortisone acetate	Cortamed, Hydrocortone Acetate	Ophthalmic	Apply a small amount to affected area 1–4 times/d

(continued)

prednisolone sodium phosphate	Inflamase, Pred Mild	Ophthalmic	1–2 drops in conjunctival sac qh during the day, then q2h at night, may decrease to 1 drop tid–qid
Nonsteroidal anti-inflammatory agents			
flurbiprofen sodium	Ansaid, Ocufen	Ophthalmic	1 drop in eye approx. q30min beginning 2 h before surgery for a total of 4 drops per affected eye
ketorolac tromethamine	Acular, Toradol	Ophthalmic	1 drop 0.5% solution qid

OTIC DRUGS

Localized ear infection or inflammation is treated by dropping a small amount of a sterile medicated solution into the ear. Conditions involving the middle or inner ear require systemic treatment. Topical ear treatmenis are most commonly used for impacted earwax and minor infections or irritation of the external ear canal.

Remember...

The use of eardrops is usually contraindicated if the patient has a perforated eardrum.

DIGESTIVE SYSTEM

The digestive tract is the organ system primarily responsible for food absorption and elimination of solid waste.

NUTRITIONAL PRODUCTS

Vitamins and minerals are essential compounds for specific body functions, such as:

- Growth
- Maintenance
- Reproduction

VITAMINS

Vitamins have no energy value, but are required for the metabolism of fats, carbohydrates, and proteins. Various amounts are needed for:

- Growing children
- Elderly people
- Pregnant women
- Lactating women

Vitamins are classified into two groups:

- Fat-soluble
- Water-soluble

The fat-soluble vitamins include:

- A (Retinol)
- D (Calciferol)
- E (Alpha-tocopherol)
- K (Phytonadione)

The water-soluble vitamins include vitamin C and the B complex vitamins. These vitamins are also called:

- Vitamin B1 = Thiamine
- Vitamin B2 = Riboflavin
- Vitamin B3 = Niacin = Nicotinic acid
- Vitamin B5 = Pantothenic acid

- Vitamin B6 = Pyridoxine
- Vitamin B9 = Folic acid
- Vitamin B12 = Cyanocobalamin
- Vitamin C = Ascorbic acid

MINERALS

Minerals are inorganic solid substances, usually occurring as part of the earth's crust. Minerals are needed for enzymes, hormones, and vitamins. They are vital for the following functions:

- Muscle contraction
- Nerve conduction
- Water balance
- Acid and base balance

Minerals are subdivided into two classes: major elements and trace elements. This classification is based on body needs, and not on importance. They may also be called **macronutrients** and **micronutrients**. The following minerals are essential for body functions:

- Iron
- Calcium
- Phosphorus
- Magnesium
- Sodium
- Potassium
- Chlorine
- Zinc
- Fluoride
- Iodine

APPENDIX A

Professional Organizations

American Association of Colleges of Pharmacy (AACP)
1426 Prince Street
Alexandria, VA 22314
(703) 739-2330
http://www.aacp.org
Established in 1900, the AACP represents all 92 pharmacy colleges and schools in the United States.

American Association of Pharmaceutical Scientists (AAPS)
2107 Wilson Blvd.
Suite 700
Arlington, VA 22201-3042
(703) 243-2800
http://www.aaps.org
Established in 1986, the AAPS provides an international forum for the exchange of knowledge among scientists to enhance their contributions to public health. The AAPS publishes the following journals: *Pharmaceutical Research*, *Pharmaceutical Development and Technology*, *AAPSPharmSciTech*, and *The AAPS Journal*.

American Association of Pharmacy Technicians (AAPT)
PO Box 1447
Greensboro, NC 27402
(877) 368-4771
http://www.pharmacytechnician.com
Established in 1979, the AAPT promotes the safe, efficacious, and cost-effective dispensing, distribution, and use of medicines.

American College of Clinical Pharmacy (ACCP)
3101 Broadway
Suite 650
Kansas City, MO 64111
(816) 531-2177
http://www.accp.com
Established in 1979, the ACCP is a professional, scientific society that provides leadership, education, advocacy, and resources that enable clinical pharmacists to achieve excellence in practice and research.

American Council on Pharmaceutical Education (ACPE)
20 North Clark Street
Suite 2500
Chicago, IL 60602-5109
(312) 664-3575
http://www.acpe-accredit.org
Also referred to as the Accreditation Council on Pharmaceutical Education, the ACPE was established in 1932 and is the national agency for the accreditation of professional degree programs in pharmacy and of providers of continuing pharmacy education.

American Pharmacists Association (APhA)
1100 15th Street NW
Suite 400
Washington, DC 20005-1707
(800) 237-2742
http://www.aphanet.org
Established in 1852 as the American Pharmaceutical Association, the APhA is a leader in providing professional education and information for pharmacists and is an advocate for improved health of the American public through the provision of comprehensive pharmaceutical care. The APhA consists of three academies:

- The Academy of Pharmacy Practice and Management (APhA-APPM)
- The Academy of Pharmaceutical Research and Science (APhA-APRS)
- The Academy of Students of Pharmacy (APhA-APS)

American Society of Health-System Pharmacists (ASHP)
7272 Wisconsin Avenue
Bethesda, MD 20814
(301) 657-3000
http://www.ashp.org
Established in 1942, the ASHP believes that the mission of pharmacists is to help people make the best use of medications. They strive to assist pharmacists in fulfilling this mission. The ASHP represents pharmacists who practice in:

- Hospitals
- Health maintenance organizations (HMOs)

- Long-term care facilities
- Home care agencies
- Other institutions

Pharmacy Technician Certification Board (PTCB)
2215 Constitution Avenue NW
Washington, DC 20037-2985
(202) 429-7576
http://www.ptcb.org
Established in 1941, the PTCB develops, maintains, promotes, and administers a high-quality certification and recertification program for pharmacy technicians.

Pharmacy Technician Educators Council (PTEC)
20122 Cabrillo Lane
Cerritos, CA 90703
(562) 860-1927, Extension 417
http://www.rxptec.org
Established in 1991, the PTEC strives to assist the profession of pharmacy in preparing high-quality, well-trained personnel through education and practical training.

United States Pharmacopoeia (USP)
12601 Twinbrook Parkway
Rockville, MD 20852-1790
(800) 227-8772
http://www.usp.org
Established in 1820, the USP is the official public standards-setting authority for all prescription and over-the-counter medications, dietary supplements, and other health-care products manufactured and sold in the United States.

National Pharmacy Technicians Association (NPTA)
PO Box 683148
Houston, TX 77268
(888) 247-8700
http://www.pharmacytechnician.org
Established in 1991, the NPTA serves to provide education, advocacy, and support to pharmacy technicians.

APPENDIX B

Professional Journals

Pharmaceutical Research
5515 Security Lane
Room 1023
Rockville, MD 20852
(301) 443-5149
http://www.pharmres.org
Pharmaceutical Research publishes innovative research papers that span the entire science spectrum that is the foundation of drug discovery, development, evaluation, and regulatory approval.

Pharmaceutical Development and Technology (Taylor & Francis Group)
325 Chestnut Street
Suite 800
Philadelphia, PA 19106
(800) 354-1420
http://www.tandf.co.uk
This journal explores the research, design, development, manufacture, and evaluation of traditional and novel drug delivery. The journal places an emphasis on practical solutions and applications to theoretical and research-based problems.

AAPSPharmSciTech
2107 Wilson Boulevard
Suite 700
Arlington, VA 22201
(703) 243-2800
http://www.aapspharmscitech.org
The mission of this online-only journal is to disseminate scientific and technical information on drug product design, development, evaluation, and processing to the global pharmaceutical research community.

The AAPS Journal
2107 Wilson Boulevard
Suite 700
Arlington, VA 22201
(703) 243-2800
http://www.aapsj.org
This peer-reviewed, online-only journal covers all areas of pharmaceutical research, including drug discovery, development, and therapy.

Today's Technician
PO Box 683148
Houston, TX 77268
(888) 247-8700
http://www.pharmacytechnician.org—Click on "magazine" to get to *Today's Technician*.
The magazine is geared specifically to the pharmacy technician and includes content on continuing education opportunities and current issues relevant to the pharmacy technician practice.

State Boards of Pharmacy

National Association of Boards of Pharmacy
Carmen A. Catizone, Executive Director
1600 Feehanville Drive
Mount Prospect, IL 60056
(847) 391-4406
http://www.nabp.net

Alabama
Jerry Moore, RPh, Exec. Dir.
10 Inverness Center, Suite 110
Birmingham, AL 35242
(205) 981-2280
rphbham@bellsouth.net
http://www.albop.com

Alaska
Barbara Roche, Licensing Examiner
PO Box 110806
Juneau, AK 99811-0806
(907) 465-2589
http://www.state.ak.us
1. Click on "Alaska State Departments."
2. Click on "Commerce, Community & Economic Development."

3. Click on "Division of Corporations, Business and Professional Licensing."
4. Click on "Boards and Commissions."
5. Click on "Pharmacy, Board of."

Arizona
Llyn A. Lloyd, RPh, Exec. Dir.
4425 W Olive Avenue, Suite 140
Glendale, AZ 85302
(623) 463-2727
vsevilla@azsbp.com
http://www.pharmacy.state.az.us

Arkansas
Charles S. Campbell, Exec. Dir.
101 E Capitol, Suite 218
Little Rock, AR 72201
(501) 682-0190
Charlie.campbell@arkansas.gov
http://www.state.ar.us

California
Patricia Harris, Exec. Officer
1625 N Market Blvd., Suite N219
Sacramento, CA 95834
(916) 574-7900
patricia_harris@dca.ca.gov
http://www.pharmacy.ca.gov

Colorado
Susan L. Warren, Program Admin.
1560 Broadway, Suite 1350
Denver, CO 80202
(303) 894-7800

pharmacy@dora.state.co.us
http://www.dora.state.co.us

Connecticut
Michelle Sylvestre, Drug Control Agent and
Board Admin.
165 Capital Avenue
Hartford, CT 06106
(860) 713-6065
Michelle.Sylvestre@po.state.ct.us
http://www.ct.gov

1. Click on "Executive."
2. Click on "Consumer Protection, Department of."
3. Click on "Boards and Commissions."
4. Click on "About the Pharmacy Commission."

Delaware
David W. Dryden, RPh, Esq.
Exec. Secretary
861 Silver Lake Blvd., Suite 203
Dover, DE 19904
(302) 744-4500
gbunting@state.de.us
http://www.professionallicensing.state.de.us—Click
on "Pharmacy."

District of Columbia
Graphelia Ramseeur, Health Licensing Specialist
825 N Capitol Street, N.E.
Washington, DC 20002
(202) 671-5000
http://dchealth.dc.gov

Florida
John D. Taylor, RPh, Exec. Dir.
4042 Bald Cypress Way
Tallahassee, FL 32399-7017
(850) 488-0595
Mqa_pharmacy@doh.state.fl.us
http://www.doh.state.fl.us—Click on "Drugs, Devices
& Cosmetics."

Georgia
Anita O. Martin, Exec. Dir.
237 Coliseum Drive
Macon, GA 31217-3858
(478) 207-2440
http://www.sos.state.ga.us
1. Click on "Professional Licensure."
2. Click on "Pharmacists."

Hawaii
Lee Ann Teshima, Exec. Officer
DCCA-PVL, Attn: PHAR
PO Box 3469
Honolulu, HI 96801
(808) 586-2694
pharmacy@dcca.state.hi.us
http://www.hawaii.gov
1. Click on "Government."
2. Click on "Functional Areas."
3. Click on "Professional and Vocational
   Licensing (PVL)."
4. Click on "Boards."
5. Click on "Pharmacy and Pharmacist."

Idaho

R.K. Markuson, RPh, Exec. Dir.
3380 Americana Terrace, Suite 320
Boise, ID 83706
(208) 334-2356
http://www.state.id.us

Illinois

Judy Cullen, Pharmacy Coord.
320 W Washington
Springfield, IL 62786
(217) 785-0800
http://www.dpr.state.il.us

Indiana

Joshua Bolin, Dir.
402 W Washington Street, Room W072
Indianapolis, IN 46204
(317) 234-2067
Hpb4@hpb.state.in.us
http://www.in.gov

1. Click on "Boards and Commissions."
2. Click on "Indiana State Board of Pharmacy."

Iowa

Lloyd K. Jessen, RPh, JD, Exec. Secretary/Dir.
400 SW 8th Street, Suite E
Des Moines, IA 50309-4633
(515) 281-5944
Debbie.Jorgensen@ibpe.state.ia.us
http://www.state.ia.us

Kansas

Susan Linn, Exec. Dir.
900 SW Jackson Street, Room 560
Topeka, KS 66612-1231
(785) 296-4056
pharmacy@ink.org
http://www.kansas.gov

1. Click on "Government."
2. Click on "Agency Web Site Listing."
3. Click on "Pharmacy, Kansas Board of."

Kentucky

Michael A. Mone, RPh, JD, Exec. Dir.
2624 Research Park Drive, Suite 302
Lexington, KY 40511
(859) 246-2820
Pharmacy.board@mail.state.ky.us
http://pharmacy.ky.gov

Louisiana

Malcolm J. Broussard, Exec. Dir.
5615 Corporate Blvd., Suite 8-E
Baton Rouge, LA 70808
(225) 925-6496
http://www.labp.com

Maine

Geraldine Betts, Board Admin.
35 State House Station
Augusta, ME 04333-0035
(207) 624-8600
Kelly.l.mclaughlin@state.me.us
http://www.maineprofessionalreg.org

Maryland
LaVerne George Nasea, Exec. Dir.
4201 Patterson Avenue
Baltimore, MD 21215-2299
(410) 764-4755
mdbop@dhmh.state.md.us
http://www.dhmh.state.md.us

Massachusetts
Charles R. Young, Exec. Dir.
239 Causeway Street, 2nd Floor, Suite 200
Boston, MA 02114
(800) 414-0168
Charles.r.young@state.ma.us
http://www.mass.gov
1. Click on "Government."
2. Click on "Branches and Departments."
3. Click on "Alphabetical List all Agencies."
4. Click on "Health and Human Services, Office of."
5. Click on "Provider."
6. Click on "Certification, Licensure and Registration."
7. Click on "Occupational and Professional."

Michigan
Melanie Brim, Licensing Mgr.
611 W Ottawa Street, 1st Floor
Lansing, MI 48933
(517) 335-0918
http://www.michigan.gov
1. Click on "Departments and Agencies."
2. Click on "Community Health."

3. Click on "Health Systems and Health Profession Licensing."
4. Click on "Licensing for Health Care Professionals."
5. Click on "Pharmacy."

Minnesota
David E. Homstrom, RPh, JD, Exec. Dir.
2829 University Avenue SE, Suite 530
Minneapolis, MN 55414-3251
(612) 617-2201
David.holmstrom@state.mn.us
http://www.phcybrd.state.mn.us

Mississippi
Leland McDivitt, Exec. Dir.
204 Key Drive, Suite D
Madison, MS 39110
(601) 605-5388
http://www.mbp.state.ms.us

Missouri
Kevin E. Kinkade, RPh, Exec. Dir.
3605 Missouri Blvd.
PO Box 625
Jefferson City, MO 65102-0625
(573) 751-0091
kkinkade@mail.state.mo.us
http://pr.mo.gov

1. Click on drop down by board "Pharmacy."

Montana

Rebecca Deschamps, RPh, Exec. Dir.
301 South Park, 4th Floor
PO Box 200513
Helena, MT 59620-0513
(406) 841-2371
dlibspdha@state.mt.us
http://mt.gov

1. Click on "State Agencies."
2. Click on "Labor and Industry Department."
3. Click on "Agency Divisions-Business Standards."
4. Click on "Permit/License Information-Healthcare Licenses."
5. Click on drop down menu "Pharmacy."

Nebraska

Becky Wisell, Exec. Secretary
PO Box 95044
Lincoln, NE 68509-5044
(402) 471-2306
http://www.hhs.state.ne.us

Nevada

Keith W. MacDonald, RPh, Exec. Secretary,
555 Double Eagle Court, #1100
Reno, NV 89521
(775) 850-1440
pharmacy@govmail.state.nv.us
http://bop.nv.gov

New Hampshire

Paul G. Boisseau, RPh, Exec. Dir.
57 Regional Drive

Concord, NH 03301
(603) 271-2350
nhpharmacy@nhsa.state.nh.us
http://www.state.nh.us

New Jersey
Debora C. Whipple, Exec. Dir.
124 Halsey Street
Newark, NJ 07102
(973) 504-6200
askconsumeraffairs@dca.lps.state.nj.us
http://www.nj.gov

1. Click on "Government Information, NJ State
   Government."
2. Click on "Departments/Agencies."
3. Click on "Attorney General/Office of:
   Department of Law & Public Safety."
4. Click on drop-down "Consumer Affairs."
5. Click on "Consumer Affairs A–Z List."
6. Click on "Pharmacists."

New Mexico
Jerry Montoya, Chief Inspector/Dir.
5200 Oakland NE, Suite A
Albuquerque, NM 87113
(505) 222-9830
Joseph.Montoya@state.nm.us
http://www.state.nm.us

New York
Lawrence H. Mokhiber, RPh, Exec. Secretary
Office of the Professions
State Education Building, 2nd Floor

Albany, NY 12234
(518) 474-3817 Extension 130
http://www.op.nysed.gov

1. Click on "List of Professions."
2. Click on "Pharmacy."

North Carolina

David R. Work, RPh, Exec. Dir.
6015 Farrington Road, Suite 201
Chapel Hill, NC 27517
(919) 246-1050
drw@ncbop.org
http://www.ncbop.org

North Dakota

Howard C. Anderson, Jr., RPh, Exec. Dir.
PO Box 1354
Bismarck, ND 58502-1354
(701) 328-9535
ndboph@btinet.net
http://www.nodakpharmacy.com

Ohio

William T. Windsley, Exec. Dir.
77 South High Street, Room 1702
Columbus, OH 43215-6126
(614) 466-4143
exec@bop.state.oh.us
http://www.state.oh.us

Oklahoma

Bryan H. Potter, RPh, Exec. Dir.
4545 Lincoln Blvd., Suite 112
Oklahoma City, OK 73105-3488

(405) 521-3815
pharmacy@oklaosf.state.ok.us
http://www.pharmacy.state.ok.us

Oregon
Gary A. Schnabel, Exec. Dir.
800 NE Oregon Street, Suite 150
Portland, OR 97232-2162
(971) 673-0001
Pharmacy.board@state.or.us
http://www.pharmacy.state.or.us

Pennsylvania
Melanie Zimmerman, Exec. Secretary
PO Box 2649
Harrisburg, PA 17105-2649
(717) 783-7156
pharmacy@pados.dos.state.pa.us
http://www.dos.state.pa.us

1. Click on "Licensing."
2. Click on "Health Related Boards."
3. Click on "Pharmacy."

Puerto Rico
Magda Bouet Grana, Exec. Dir.
Call Box 10200
Santurce, PR 00908
(787) 725-8161
mbouet@salud.gov.pr
http://www.salud.gov.pr

Rhode Island
Catherine A. Cordy, Chief of the Board
3 Capitol Hill
Providence, RI 02908
(401) 222-2231
dianet@doh.state.ri.us
http://www.health.ri.gov

South Carolina
LeeAnn Bundrick, Interim Admin.
110 Centerview Drive
Columbia, SC 29210
(803) 896-4700
funderbm@mail.llr.state.sc.us
http://www.llr.state.sc.us

South Dakota
Dennis M. Jones, RPh, Exec. Secretary
4305 S Louise Avenue, Suite 104
Sioux Falls, SD 57106-3115
(605) 362-2737
Dennis.jones@state.sd.us
http://www.state.sd.us

Tennessee
Kendall M. Lynch, Dir.
500 James Robertson Pkwy., 2nd Floor
Nashville, TN 37243-1149
(615) 741-2718
klynch@mail.state.tn.us
http://www.state.tn.us

Texas

Gay Dodson, RPh, Exec. Dir.
333 Guadalupe Street, Tower 3, Suite 600
Austin, TX 78701
(512) 305-8000
geninfo@tsbp.state.tx.us
http://www.tsbp.state.tx.us

Utah

Diana L. Baker, Bureau Dir.
160 E 300 South
Salt Lake City, UT 84111
(801) 530-6628
dbaker@utah.gov
http://www.dopl.utah.gov

Vermont

Peggy Atkins, Board Admin.
PO Box 70
108 Cherry Street
Burlington, VT 05402
(802) 657-4220
cpreston@sec.state.vt.us
http://www.vtprofessionals.org

Virgin Islands

Lydia T. Scott, Exec. Asst.
Roy L. Schneider Hospital
St. Thomas, VI 00802
(340) 774-0117
Lydia.scott@usvi-doh.org
http://www.usvi.org

Virginia
Elizabeth Scott Russell, RPh, Exec. Dir.
6603 W Broad Street, 5th Floor
Richmond, VA 23230-1712
(804) 662-9911
Scotti.Russell@dhp.state.va.us
http://www.dhp.state.va.us

Washington
Donald H. Williams, RPh, Exec. Dir.
310 Israel Road
Tumwater, WA 98501
(360) 236-4700
Don.Williams@doh.wa.gov
https://fortress.wa.gov

West Virginia
William T. Douglass, Jr., Exec. Dir.
232 Capitol Street
Charleston, WV 25301
(304) 558-0558
wdouglass@wvbop.com
http://www.wvbop.com

Wisconsin
Deanna Zychowski, Dir.
PO Box 8935
Madison, WI 53708-8935
(608) 266-2112
web@drl.state.wi.us
http://www.state.wi.us

Wyoming

James T. Carder, Exec. Dir.
632 S David Street
Casper, WY 82601
(307) 234-0294
wypharmbd@wercs.com
http://pharmacyboard.state.wy.us

APPENDIX D

Converting Measurements

LENGTH	Centimeters	Inches	Feet
1 centimeter	1.000	0.394	0.0328
1 inch	2.54	1.000	0.0833
1 foot	30.48	12.000	1.000
1 yard	91.4	36.00	3.00
1 meter	100.00	39.40	3.28

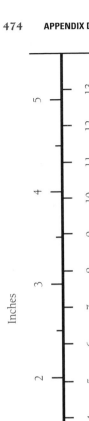

VOLUMES	Cubic Centimeters	Fluid Drams	Fluid Ounces	Quarts	Liters
1 cubic centimeter	1.00	0.270	0.033	0.0010	0.0010
1 fluid dram	3.70	1.00	0.125	0.0039	0.0037
1 cubic inch	16.39	4.43	0.554	0.0173	0.0163
1 fluid ounce	29.6	8.00	1.000	0.0312	0.0296
1 quart	946.0	255.0	32.00	1.000	0.946
1 liter	1000.0	270.0	33.80	1.056	1.000

WEIGHTS	Grains	Grams	Apothecary Ounces	Pounds
1 grain (gr)	1.000	0.064	0.002	0.0001
1 gram (gm)	15.43	1.000	0.032	0.0022
1 apothecary ounce	480.00	31.1	1.000	0.0685
1 pound	7000.00	454.0	14.58	1.000
1 kilogram	15432.0	1000.00	32.15	2.205

RULES FOR CONVERTING ONE SYSTEM TO ANOTHER

VOLUMES

Grains to grams—divide by 15
Drams to cubic centimeters—multiply by 4
Ounces to cubic centimeters—multiply by 30
Minims to cubic millimeters—multiply by 63
Minims to cubic centimeters—multiply by 0.06
Cubic millimeters to minims—divide by 63
Cubic centimeters to minims—multiply by 16
Cubic centimeters to fluid ounces—divide by 30
Liters to pints—divide by 2

WEIGHTS

Milligrams to grains—multiply by 0.0154
Grams to grains—multiply by 15
Grams to drams—multiply by 0.257
Grams to ounces—multiply by 0.0311

TEMPERATURE

Multiply centigrade (Celsius) degrees by $\frac{9}{5}$ and add 32 to convert Fahrenheit to Celsius.

Subtract 32 from the Fahrenheit degrees and multiply by $\frac{9}{5}$ to convert Celsius to Fahrenheit.

COMMON HOUSEHOLD MEASURES AND WEIGHTS

1 teaspoon	=	4–5 cc. or 1 dram
3 teaspoons	=	1 tablespoon
1 dessert spoon	=	8 cc. or 2 drams
1 tablespoon	=	15 cc. or 3 drams
4 tablespoons	=	1 wineglass or $\frac{1}{2}$ gill
6 tablespoons (liq)	=	1 cup
2 tablespoons (dry)	=	1 cup
1 cup	=	8 fluid ounces or $\frac{1}{2}$ pint
1 tumbler or glass	=	8 fluid ounces or 240 cc.
1 wineglass	=	2 fluid ounces, 60 cc.
6 fluid ounces	=	1 pound
4 gills	=	1 pound
1 pint	=	1 pound

APPENDIX E

Medical Symbols and Abbreviations

m	minim	⁻s	without
ʒ	dram	⁻c	with
ʒ	ounce	−	minus, negative, alkaline reaction
O	pint	+	plus, excess, acid reaction, positive
#	pound, number		
℞	recipe, prescription		
'	foot, minute	×	multiply
"	inch, second	÷	divide
a̅a̅	equal parts	=	equals
°	degree	>	greater than
%	percent	<	less than
♂	male	∞	infinity
♀	female	↑	increase
s̅s̅	one half	↓	decrease

The Most Common Poisonous Substances and Their Antidotes

Drug	Antidote
Acetaminophen	Acetylcystein
eAnticholinesterases (cholinergics)	Atropine, pralidoxime
Antidepressants (MAO inhibitors and tyramine-containing foods)	Phentolamine
Benzodiazepines	Flumazenil
Cyanide	Amyl nitrite, sodium nitrite, sodium thiosulfate
Digoxin, digitoxin	Digoxin immune Fab (Digibind)
Fluorouracil (5FU)	Leucovorin calcium
Heparin	Protamine sulfate
Ifosfamide	Mesna
Iron	Deferoxamine

(continued)

Lead	Edentate calcium disodium, dimercaprol, succimer
Methotrexate	Leucovorin calcium
Opioid analgesics, heroin	Nalmefene, naloxone
Thrombolytic agents	Aminocaproic acid (Amicar)
Tricyclic antidepressants	Physostigmine
Warfarin (Coumadin)	Phytonadione (vitamin K)

APPENDIX G

The Most Commonly Prescribed Drugs in 2005

(These drugs are listed in descending order beginning with the most prescribed drug, hydrocodone w/APAP.)

Generic Name	Brand Name
hydrocodone w/APAP	Hydrocodone w/APAP
atorvastatin	Lipitor
atenolol	Tenormin
levothyroxine	Synthroid
conjugated estrogens	Premarin
azithromycin	Zithromax
furosemide	Lasix
amoxicillin	Amoxil
amlodipine	Norvasc
hydrochlorothiazide	Hydro-Diuril
alprazolam	Xanax
albuterol	Proventil, Ventolin
sertraline hydrochloride	Zoloft
paroxetine hydrochloride	Paxil

(continued)

simvastatin	Zocor
lansoprazole	Prevacid
ibuprofen	Motrin, Advil, Nuprin
triamterene	Dyrenium
metoprolol succinate	Toprol-XL
cephalexin monohydrate	Keflex
celecoxib	Celebrex
cetirizine hydrochloride	Zyrtec
levothyroxine sodium	Levoxyl
fexofenadine hydrochloride	Allegra
norgestimate/ethinyl estradiol	Ortho Evra
citalopram hydrobromide	Celexa
prednisone	Deltasone
omeprazole	Prilosec
loratadine	Claritin
fluoxetine hydrochloride	Prozac
acetaminophen	Tylenol
zolpidem tartrate	Ambien
metoprolol tartrate	Lopressor
lorazepam	Ativan
alendronate sodium	Fosamax
propoxyphene N/APAP	Darvon-N
metformin hydrochloride	Glucophage, Fortamet

(continued)

ranitidine hydrochloride	Zantac
amitriptyline hydrochloride	Elavil
sildenafil citrate	Viagra
conjugated estrogens/ medroxyprogesterone	Prempro
amoxicillin	Trimox
gabapentin	Neurontin
bupropion HCL	Wellbutrin SR
pravastatin sodium	Pravachol
amoxicillin/clavulanate	Augmentin
esomeprazole	Nexium
quinapril hydrochloride	Accupril
lisinopril	Prinivil, Zestril
venlafaxine	Effexor XR
montelukast sodium	Singulair
lisinopril	Zestril
potassium chloride	Potassium chloride, (K-Lease), Klorvess
clonazepam	Klonopin
naproxen	Naprosyn
warfarin sodium	Coumadin
trazodone hydrochloride	Desyrel
ciprofloxacin hydrochloride	Cipro
fluticasone propionate	Flonase

(continued)

cyclobenzaprine hydrochloride	Flexeril
verapamil	Calan, Isoptin
enalapril maleate	Vasotec
isosorbide mononitrate	Ismo, Imdur
levofloxacin	Levaquin
diazepam	Valium
glipizide	Glucotrol XL
warfarin	Coumadin
clopidogrel bisulfate	Plavix
fluconazole	Diflucan
salmeterol/xinafoate	Serevent Diskus
pantoprazole sodium	Protonix
amlodipine	Norvasc
valsartan	Diovan
glyburide	Micronase
ramipril	Altace
allopurinol	Allopurinol Zyloprim
estradiol	EstroGel
rosiglitazone maleate	Avandia
pioglitazone hydrochloride	Actos
benazepril hydrochloride	Lotensin
desloratadine	Clarinex
medroxyprogesterone acetate	Depo-Provera C-150, Provera

(continued)

oxycodone hydrochloride	Roxicodone
doxycycline hyclate	Vibramycin
digoxin	Lanoxin
losartan potassium	Cozaar
mometasone furoate	Nasonex
diltiazem hydrochloride	ardizem
clonidine hydrochloride	Catapres
digoxin	Digitek
methylprednisolone	Medrol
raloxifene hydrochloride	Evista
folic acid	Folvite
metformin hydrochloride	Glucophage XR
penicillin V Potassium	Penicillin VK
risperidone	Risperdal
trimethoprimsulfamethoxazole	Septra
valsartan	Diovan
rabeprazole sodium	Aciphex
olanzapine	Zyprexa
levothyroxine sodium	Levothroid
doxazosin mesylate	Cardura
latanoprost	Xalatan
gemfibrozil	Lopid
tamsulosin hydrochloride	Flomax

(continued)

temazepam	Restoril
tramadol hydrochloride	Ultram
isophane insulin suspension	Humulin N
divalproex sodium	Depakote
methylphenidate hydrochloride	Concerta
glyburide	Micronase
sumatriptan succinate	Imitrex
terazosin	Hytrin
loratadine	Claritin
glimepiride	Amaryl
spironolactone	Aldactrone
fenofibrate	Tricor
norethindrone/ethinyl estradiol	Ortho-Novum
hydroxyzine hydrochloride	Atarax, Vistaril
fosinopril sodium	Monopril
ipratropium/albuterol	Combivent
meclizine hydrochloride	Antivert
triamcinolone acetonide	Kenalog, Aristocart
metoclopramide	Reglan, Maxdon
bisoprolol fumorate	Zebeta
propranolol hydrochloride	Inderal
propoxyphene hydrochloride	Darvon
valacyclovir hydrochloride	Valtrex

(continued)

mirtazapine	Remeron
famotidine	Pepcid
metronidazole	Flagyl
irbesartan	Avapro
glipizide	Glucotrol
buspirone hydrochloride	BuSpar
nystatin	Mycostatin, Nilstat, Nystex
phenytoin	Dilantin
ethinyl estradiol/norethindrone	Necon
captopril	Capoten
clindamycin hydrochloride	Cleocin
aspirin	Bayer
quetiapine fumarate	Seroquel
acyclovir	Zovirax
amoxicillin potassium clavulanate	Augmentin
amphetamine mixed salts	Adderall XR
clarithromycin	Biaxin
levonorgestrel/ethinyl estradiol	Trivora-28
norgestimate/ethinyl estradiol	Ortho-Cyclen
cefprozil	Cefzil
isophane insulin suspension	Humulin 70/30
tolterodine titrate	Detrol LA

(continued)

carvedilol	Coreg
diltiazem hydrochloride	Tiazac
tramadol hydrochloride	Ultram
insulin lispro	Humalog
oxycodone/APAP	Endocet
mupirocin	Bactroban
penicillin V potassium	Veetids
timolol maleate	Blocadren, Timoptic, Betimol
budesonide	Rhinocort
nortriptyline hydrochloride	Aventyl
levonorgestrel/ethinyl estradiol	Aviane
risedronate sodium	Actonel
topiramate	Topamax
norethindrone/ethinyl estradiol	Microgestin Fe
tamoxifen	Nolvadex
desogestrel/ethinyl estradiol	Mircette
nifedipine	Adalat, Procardia
tetracycline hydrochloride	Sumycin
desogestrel/ethinyl estradiol	Apri
diclofenac sodium	Voltaren
carbidopa/levodopa	Sinemet
azelastine hydrochloride	Astelin

APPENDIX H

Controlled Substances in the United States and Canada

CONTROLLED SUBSTANCES ACT—UNITED STATES

The U.S. Federal Controlled Substances Act of 1970 placed drugs controlled by the Act into five categories, or schedules, based on their potential to cause psychological and/or physical dependence as well as on their potential for abuse. The schedules are defined as follows:

- **Schedule I [C-I]:** Includes substances for which there is a high abuse potential and no current approved medical use (for example, heroin, marijuana, LSD, other hallucinogens, certain opiates, and opium derivatives).

Note: Marijuana has recently been approved for specific medical use in certain states, but is still considered a Schedule I drug.

- **Schedule II [C-II]:** Includes drugs that have a high ability to produce physical or psychological dependence and for which there is a current approved or acceptable medical use (for example, narcotics, certain CNS stimulants).

- **Schedule III [C-III]:** Includes drugs for which there is less potential for abuse than drugs in Schedule II and for which there is a current approved medical use and moderate dependence liability. Certain drugs in this category are preparations containing limited quantities of codeine and non-barbiturate sedatives. Anabolic steroids are classified in Schedule III.

- **Schedule IV [C-IV]:** Includes drugs for which there is less abuse potential than for Schedule III, for which there is a current approved medical use, and that have limited dependence liability (for example, some sedatives, antianxiety drugs, non-narcotic analgesics).

- **Schedule V [C-V]:** Drugs in this category have limited abuse potential and consist mainly of preparations containing limited amounts of certain narcotic drugs for use as antitussives and antidiarrheals. Federal law provides that an individual at least 18 years of age may purchase limited quantities of these drugs (for example, codeine) without a prescription if allowed under state statutes. The product must be purchased from a pharmacist, who in turn must keep appropriate records. However, state laws vary, and in many states such products require a prescription.

Note: Generally, prescriptions for Schedule II (high abuse potential) drugs cannot be transmitted over the phone and they cannot be refilled. Prescriptions for Schedule III, IV, and V drugs may be refilled up to five times within six months. Schedule II drugs are not necessarily "stronger" than drugs in Schedules III, IV, or V; Schedule II drugs are classified as such due to their high abuse potential. Drugs that are not controlled are indicated by an asterisk (*).

CONTROLLED SUBSTANCES—CANADA

In Canada, there are eight schedules. They are:

I. Some of the more common groups include opium derivatives and salts (for example, codeine, morphine, hydrocodone, oxycodone, oxymorphone); coca derivatives and salts (for example, cocaine); phenylpiperidines and derivatives and salts (for example, difenoxin, diphenoxylate, pethidine); phenazepines and salts (for example, ethoheptazine); amidones and salts (for example, methadone); phenalkoxams and salts (for example, dextropropoxyphene); morphinans and salts (for example, buprenorphine, levorphanol); benzazocines and salts (for example, pentazocine); phencyclidine and salts; and fentanyls and salts (alfentanil, fentanyl, remifentanil, sufentanil). (*Note*: The preceding Schedule I list is not inclusive.)

II. Cannabis and derivatives (for example, marijuana, cannabinol).

III. Amphetamines, their salts, and derivatives (for example, amphetamine, benzphetamine). Also, methylphenidate, psilocin, psilocybin, and mescaline.

IV. Barbiturates and their salts and thiobarbiturates and salts. Also, anabolic steroids, benzodiazpines, chlorphentermine, diethylpropion, phendimetrazine, phentermine, butorphanol, nalbuphine, glutethimide, ethchlorvynol, maxindol, meprobamate, and methyprylon.

V. Phenylpropanolamine and propylhexedrine.

VI. Ephedrine, ergotamine, LSD, and pseudoephedrine.

VII. Specific amounts of cannabis (3 kg) and cannabis resin (3 kg).

VIII. Specific amounts of cannabis (30 g) and cannabis resin (1 g).

Drug Schedule

Drug	United States	Canada
Alfentanil	II	I
Alprazolam	IV	IV
Amobarbital sodium	II	IV
Amphetamine sulfate	II	III
Aprobarbital	III	IV
Benzphetamine HCl	III	III
Buprenorphine HCl	III	I
Butabarbital sodium	III	IV
Butorphanol tartrate	IV	IV
Chloral hydrate	IV	*
Chlordiazepoxide	IV	IV
Clonazepam	IV	IV

(continued)

Clorazepate dipotassium	IV	IV
Cocaine	II	I
Codeine	II	I
Dexmethylphenidate HCl	II	Not available
Dextroamphetamine sulfate	II	III

Dextropropoxyphene
  Bulk
  Dosage Forms
	
	II
	IV
		
		I
		I

Diazepam	IV	IV
Diethylpropion HCl	IV	IV
Difenoxin products (0.5 mg/25 mcg atropine sulfate)	V	I
Diphenoxylate products (2.5 mg/25 mcg atropine sulfate)	V	I
Dronabinol	III	*
Estazolam	IV	IV
Ethchlorvynol	IV	IV
Fentanyl	II	I
Fluoxymesterone	III	IV
Flurazepam HCl	IV	IV
Glutethimide	II	IV
Halazepam	IV	IV
Hydrocodone	Not available alone (usually C-III in combination drugs)	I

(*continued*)

Hydromorphone HCl	II	I
Ketamine	III	*
Levorphanol tartrate	II	I
Lorazepam	IV	IV
Mazindol	IV	IV
Meperidine HCl	II	I
Mephobarbital	IV	IV
Meprobamate	IV	IV
Methadone HCl	II	I
Methamphetamine HCl	II	III
Methandrostenolone	III	IV
Methylphenidate HCl	II	III
Methyltestosterone	III	IV
Midazolam	IV	IV
Modafinil	IV	*
Morphine sulfate	II	I
Nandrolone decanoate	III	IV
Opium	II	I
Opium products (100 mg/100 mL or gm)	V	I
Oxandrolone	III	IV
Oxazepam	IV	IV
Oxycodone HCl	II	I
Oxymetholone	III	IV

(continued)

Oxymorphone HCl	II	I
Paraldehyde	IV	*
Paregoric	III	I
Pemoline	IV	*
Pentazocine	IV	I
Pentobarbital sodium		
PO	II	IV
Rectal	III	IV
Phencyclidine	II	I
Phendimetrazine tartrate	III	IV
Phenobarbital	IV	IV
Phentermine HCl	IV	IV
Prazepam	IV	IV
Quazepam	IV	IV
Remifentanil HCl	II	–
Secobarbital sodium	II	IV
Sibutramine HCl	IV	–
Stanolone	III	IV
Stanozolol	III	IV
Sufentanil citrate	II	I
Temazepam	IV	IV
Testosterone (all forms)	III	IV
Thiopental	III	IV
Triazolam	IV	IV

(continued)

Zaleplon	IV	–
Zolpidem tartrate	IV	–

Reprinted from Spratto, G. and Woods, A. (2006) *PDR Nurse's Drug Handbook*. Thomson Delmar Learning: Clifton Park, NY.

APPENDIX I

Pregnancy Categories: FDA Assigned

The U.S. Food and Drug Administration's use-in-pregnancy rating system weighs the degree to which available information has ruled out risk to the fetus against the drug's potential benefit to the patient. The ratings and their interpretation are as follows:

Category	Interpretation
A	**Controlled studies show no risk.** Adequate, well-controlled studies in pregnant women have failed to demonstrate a risk to the fetus in any trimester of pregnancy.
B	**No evidence of risk in humans.** Either animal studies show risk, but human findings do not, or if no adequate human studies have been done, animal findings are negative.

(continued)

C   **Risk cannot be ruled out.** Human studies are lacking, and animal studies are either positive for fetal risk or lacking. However, potential benefits might justify the potential risks.

D   **Positive evidence of risk.** Investigational or post-marketing data show risk to the fetus. However, potential benefits might outweigh the potential risks. If needed in a life-threatening situation or serious disease, the drug might be acceptable if safer drugs cannot be used or are ineffective.

X   **Contraindicated in pregnancy.** Studies in animals or humans, or investigational or post-marketing reports, have demonstrated positive evidence of fetal abnormalities or risks, which clearly outweigh any possible benefit to the patient.

Reprinted from Spratto, G. and Woods, A. (2006) *PDR Nurse's Drug Handbook*. Thomson Delmar Learning: Clifton Park, NY.

APPENDIX J

Drug/Food Interactions

(See individual drug write-up.)

A. DRUGS THAT SHOULD BE TAKEN WHILE FASTING

Ampicillin

AzoGantanol/Gantrisin

Bacampicillin

Bethanechol (may experience N&V)

Bisacodyl

Calcium carbonate

Captopril

Carbenicillin

Castor oil

Chloramphenicol

Claritin

Cyclosporine gel caps only (Avoid fatty meals.)

Demeclocycline (Avoid high-calcium foods/dairy
    products.)

Dicloxacillin

Disopyramide

Digitalis preparations (Do not take with
    high-fiber foods.)

Erythromycin base/estolate

Etidronate

Ferrous salts (Do not take with tea, coffee, egg, cereals, fiber, or milk.)

Fexofenadine

Flavoxate

Furosemide

Isoniazid

Isosorbide dinitrate

Ketoprofen (If GI distress occurs, may take with food.)

Lansoprazole

Levodopa (Do not take with high-protein foods; meals delay absorption and peak plasma concentration; avoid caffeine.)

Lisinopril

Lomustil (An empty stomach will reduce nausea.)

Methotrexate (Milk, cream, or yogurt might decrease absorption.)

Methyldopa (Do not take with high-protein foods; meals delay absorption and peak plasma concentration; avoid caffeine.)

Nafcillin (Inactivated by stomach acid; absorption is variable with/without food.)

Nalidixic acid

Naltrexone

Norfloxacin (Milk, cream, or yogurt might decrease absorption.)

Oxytetracycline (Avoid dairy products and high-calcium foods.)

Penicillamine (Antacids, iron, and food decrease absorption.)

Penicillin

Phenytoin (If GI distress occurs, may take with food; food effect depends on preparation.)

Propantheline

Rifampicin

Sotalol

Sulfamethoxazole

Tetracycline (Avoid dairy products and high-calcium foods.)

Theophylline (Absorption of controlled release varies by preparation.)

Thyroid hormone preparations (Limit foods containing goitrogens.)

Terbutaline sulfate

Trientine (Antacids, iron, and food reduce absorption.)

Trimethoprim

Zyrtec

B. DRUGS THAT SHOULD BE TAKEN WITH FOOD

Buspirone

Carbamazepine (Erratic absorption.)

Chlorothiazide

Clofazimine

Gemfibrozil

Griseofulvin (Take with high-fat meals.)

Isotretinoin

Labetalol

Lovastatin

Methenamine

Metoprolol

Nifedipine (Grapefruit juice increases bioavailability.)

Nitrofurantoin

Oxcarbazepine

Probucol (Take with high-fat meals.)

Propranolol

Spironolactone

Trazodone

Verapamil SR (Absorption varies by manufacturer; too-rapid absorption might cause heart block.)

C. CONSTIPATING AGENTS

Antacids

Anticholinergic drugs

  Antihistamines

  Anticholinergics

  Phenothiazines

  Tricyclic antidepressants

Corticosteroids

Clonidine

Ganglionic blocking agents

Iron supplements

Laxatives (When abused.)

Lithium

MAO Inhibitors

Muscle relaxants

Octreotide

Opioids

Prostaglandin synthesis inhibitors
NSAIDS

D. DIARRHEAL AGENTS

Adrenergic neuron blockers: reserpine, guanethidine
Antibiotics (Especially broad-spectrum agents.)
Cholinergic agonists and cholinesterase inhibitors
Erythromycin
Glucophage
Osmotic and stimulant laxatives
Metoclopramide
Quinidine

E. TYRAMINE-CONTAINING FOODS

Moderate amounts of tyramine:

Broad beans

Raspberries

Banana peel

Cheese (all except cream cheese and cottage cheese)

Imitation cheese

Prepared meats (sausage, chopped liver, pate, salami, mortadella)

Meat extracts

Concentrated yeast extracts/Brewer's yeast

Liquid and powdered protein supplements

Fermented soy products: fermented bean curd (tofu), soybean paste (miso), miso soup

Hydrolyzed protein extracts for sauces, soups, gravies

Fermented cabbage products: sauerkraut, kimchee

Chianti, vermouth

Nonalcoholic beers

Some non-U.S. brands of beer

Significant amounts of tyramine:

Avocado

Yogurt

Cream from fresh, pasteurized milk

Soy sauce

Peanuts

Chocolate

Red and white wines, port wines

Distilled spirits

F. FOODS CONTAINING GOITROGENS

Asparagus

Brussels sprouts

Cabbage

Kale

Lettuce

Peas

Soybeans

Spinach

Turnip greens

Watercress

Other leafy green vegetables

G. COUMARIN ANTICOAGULANTS AND DIETARY EFFECTS

Consumption of vitamin K-enriched foods might counteract the effects of anticoagulants because the drugs act through antagonism of vitamin K. Advise client on anticoagulants to maintain a steady, consistent intake of vitamin K-containing foods. The drug monograph for warfarin clearly lists these foods. In addition, certain herbal teas (Woodruff, tonka beans, melitot) contain natural coumarins that can potentiate the effects of Coumadin and should be avoided. Large amounts of avocado also potentiate the drug's effects. Brussels sprouts and other cruciferous vegetables increase the catabolism of warfarin, thereby decreasing its anticoagulant activities.

H. GENERAL DRUG CLASS RECOMMENDATIONS

ACE inhibitors: Take captopril and moexipril 1 hr before or 2 hr after meals; food decreases absorption. Avoid high-potassium foods because ACE increases K+.

Analgesic/Antipyretic: Take on an empty stomach because food might slow the absorption.

Antacids: Take 1 hr after or between meals. Avoid dairy foods because the protein in them can increase stomach acid.

Anti-anxiety agents: Caffeine may cause excitability, nervousness, and hyperactivity, thus lessening the anti-anxiety drug effects.

Antibiotics: Penicillin generally should be taken on an empty stomach; it may be taken with food if GI upset occurs. Do not mix with acidic foods such as coffee, citrus fruits, and tomatoes. The acid interferes with absorption of penicillin, ampicillin, erythromycin, and cloxacillin.

Anticoagulants: High vitamin K produces a blood-clotting substance and might reduce drug effectiveness.

Vitamin E >400 IU might prolong clotting time and increase bleeding risk.

Antidepressant drugs: May be taken with or without food.

Antifungals: Avoid taking with dairy products; avoid alcohol.

Antihistamines: Take on an empty stomach to increase effectiveness.

Bronchodilators with theophylline: High-fat meals might increase bioavailability, while high-carbohydrate meals might decrease it. Food increases absorption of Theo-24 and Uniphyl, which might cause increased N&V, headache, and irritability.

Cephalosporins: Take on an empty stomach 1 hr before or 2 hr after meals. May take with food if GI upset occurs.

Diuretics: Vary in interactions. Some cause loss of potassium, calcium, and magnesium. Avoid salty food and natural black licorice because these increase K and Mg losses. Large doses of vitamin D can elevate blood pressure.

H2 blockers: May take with or without regard to food.

HMG-CoA reductase inhibitors: Take lovastatin with the evening meal to enhance absorption.

Laxatives: Avoid dairy foods because calcium can decrease absorption.

Macrolides: Take on an empty stomach 1 hr before or 2 hr after meals. May take with food for GI upset.

MAO inhibitors: Have many dietary restrictions, so follow dietary guidelines as prescribed. Foods or alcoholic beverages containing tyramine might cause a fatal increase in BP.

Narcotic analgesics: Avoid alcohol because it might increase sedative effects.

Nitroimadazole (metronidazole): Avoid alcohol or food prepared with alcohol for at least three days after finishing the medicine. Alcohol might cause nausea, abdominal cramps, vomiting, headaches, and flushing.

NSAIDS: Take with food or milk to prevent irritation of the stomach.

Quinolones: Take on an empty stomach 1 hr before or 2 hr after meals. May take with food for GI upset, but avoid calcium-containing foods such as milk, yogurt, vitamins/minerals containing iron, and antacids because they decrease drug concentrations. Caffeine-containing products might lead to excitability and nervousness.

Sulfonamides: Take on an empty stomach 1 hr before or 2 hr after meals. May take with food if GI upset occurs.

Tetracyclines: Take on an empty stomach 1 hr before or 2 hr after meals. May take with food, but avoid dairy products, antacids, and vitamins containing iron when taking tetracycline.

Reprinted from Spratto, G. and Woods, A. (2006) *PDR Nurse's Drug Handbook*. Thomson Delmar Learning: Clifton Park, NY.

APPENDIX K

Drugs that Should Not Be Crushed

As a rule of thumb, any sustained-release or extended-release formulation should never be crushed. Instead, attempt to get a liquid formulation of the product so that it can be administered in that form. Coated products also should not be crushed. They were coated for a specific purpose, for example, to prevent stomach irritation by the product, to prevent destruction of the product by stomach acid, to prevent an unwanted reaction, or to produce a prolonged or an extended effect.

Some of the drugs that should not be crushed are the following:

Accutane	ASA E.C.
aciphex	ASA enseal
adalat cc SR	augmentin XR
advicor ER	Azulfadine entab
Afrinol repetab	Betaphen-vk
Allerest capsule	Biaxin XL
Allegra D	Biscodyl EC
Aminodur duratab	Calan SR
Artane sequel	Cardiazem LS, SR
arthrotec	Ceclor DC

Ceftin
Chlortrimeton SR
Choledyl SR
Cipro XR
Claritin D
Colace
Colestid
Compazine spansule
Concerta SR
Covera hs ER
Creon EC
Depakote EC, ER
Desyrel
Dexedrine SR
Diamox sequel
Dilacor XR
Dimetapp SR
Ditropan XL
Donnatol extentab
Drixoral tablet
Ecotrin tablet
Effexor XR
E-Mycin tablet
Entex LA
Erythromycins EC
Feldene
Feosol spansule
Feosol tablet

Ferro Grad-500 tablet
Flomax
Glucophage XR
Glucatrol XL
Humibid DM, LA
Imdur SR, LA
Indocin SR
Isoptin SR
Isordil sublingual
Isordil tembids, dinatrate
Kaon tablet
K-Dur, K-tab
Klor-Con
Levbid SR
Lithobid SR
Macrobid SR
Mestinon timespnas
metadate CD, SR
MS Contin
Mucinex
Nexium
Niaspan
Nitroglycerin tablet
Nitrospan capsule
Norpace CR
Ornade spansule
OxyContin
Pancrease EC, MT

Paxil CR

Pentosa

Phazyme

Plendil SR

Prevacid

Prilosec SR

Procardia XL

Protonix

Proventil Repetabs

Prozac weekly

Quinaglute duratab

Quinidex extenutab

Slow K tablet; slow mag, slow Fe

Sorbitrate sl

Sudafed SA capsule

Tegretol XR

Teldrin capsule

Tenuate dospan

Tessalon Perles

Theobid duracaps

Theolair SR

Thorazine Spansules

TiazacSR

Toprol SL

Trental SR

Tylenol ER

Uniphyl SR

Verelan PM

Volmax SR

Voltaren EC

Voltaren SR

Wellbutrin SR

Xanax SR

Zerit XR

Zomig DR

Zyban

Zyrtec-D

Reprinted from Spratto, G. and Woods, A. (2006) *PDR Nurse's Drug Handbook*. Thomson Delmar Learning: Clifton Park, NY.

APPENDIX L

Pharmaceutical Companies

Abbott Laboratories
U.S. Corporate Headquarters
Abbott Laboratories
100 Abbott Park Road
Abbott Park, IL 60064-3500
Telephone: (847) 937-6100
http://www.abbott.com

Allergan, Inc.
PO Box 19534
Irvine, CA 92623
USA
Telephone: (714) 246-4500
Fax: (714) 246-4971
http://www.allergan.com

Amgen, Inc.
Corporate Headquarters
One Amgen Center Drive
Thousand Oaks, CA 91320-1799
Telephone: (805) 447-1000
Fax: (805) 447-1010
http://www.amgen.com

AstraZeneca Pharmaceuticals LP
U.S. Headquarters
PO Box 15437
Wilmington, DE 19850-5437
Telephone: (302) 886-3000
Fax: (302) 866-2972
http://www.astrazeneca-us.com

Bausch & Lomb
World Headquarters
One Bausch & Lomb Place
Rochester, NY 14604-2701
Telephone: (585) 338-6000
Fax: (585) 338-6007
http://www.bausch.com

Baxter International
One Baxter Parkway
Deerfield, IL 60015-4625
Telephone: (847) 948-2000
http://www.baxter.com

Bayer Corporation
Pharmaceutical Division
400 Morgan Lane
West Haven, CT 06516
Telephone: (800) 468-0894
Fax: (203) 812-2000
http://www.pharma.bayer.com

Biogen Idec
14 Cambridge Center
Cambridge, MA 02142
Telephone: (617) 679-2000

Fax: (617) 679-2617
http://www.biogenidec.com

Boehringer Ingelheim
Corporate Headquarters
Binger Street 173
55216 Ingelheim, Germany
Telephone: 49 6132-77-0
Fax: 49-6132-72-0
http://www.boehringer-ingelheim.com

Bristol-Myers Squibb
345 Park Avenue
New York, NY 10154-0037
Telephone: (212) 546-4000
http://www.bms.com

Chiron Corporation (See Novartis)

Eli Lilly and Company
Lilly Corporate Center
Indianapolis, IN 46285
Telephone: (317) 276-2000
http://www.lilly.com

Forest Laboratories
Corporate Headquarters
909 Third Avenue
New York, NY 10022
Telephone: (212) 421-7850 or (800) 947-5227
http://www.frx.com

Genentech, Inc.
Corporate Headquarters
1 DNA Way

South San Francisco, CA 94080-4990
Telephone: (650) 225-1000
Fax: (650) 225-6000
http://www.gene.com

Genzyme
Corporate Offices
500 Kendall Street
Cambridge, MA 02142
Telephone: (617) 252-7500
Fax: (617) 252-7600
http://www.genzyme.com

GlaxoSmithKline
1 Franklin Plaza
PO Box 7929
Philadelphia, PA 19101-7929
Telephone: (888) 825-5249
http://www.gsk.com

Hoffman-La Roche
Corporate Headquarters
Grezacherstrasse 124
CH-4070 Basel
Switzerland
Telephone: 41-61-688-1111
Fax: 41-61-691-9391
http://www.roche.com

Johnson & Johnson
One Johnson & Johnson Plaza
New Brunswick, NJ 08933
Telephone: (732) 524-0400
http://www.jnj.com

Merck & Co., Inc.
One Merck Drive
PO Box 100
Whitehouse Station, NJ 08889-0100
Telephone: (908) 423-1000
http://www.merck.com

Novartis
(Formerly Chiron Corporation)
4560 Horton Street
Emeryville, CA 94608-2916
Telephone: (510) 655-8730
Fax: (510) 655-9910
http://www.chiron.com or http://www.norvartis.com

Novo Nordisk, Inc.
100 College Road West
Princeton, NJ 08540
Telephone: (866) 668-6336
http://www.novonordisk-us.com

Pfizer, Inc.
235 East 42nd Street
New York, NY 10017
Telephone: (212) 733-2323
http://www.pfizer.com

Proctor & Gamble
One P & G Plaza
Cincinnati, OH 45202
Telephone: (866) 776-2837
http://www.pg.com

sanofi-aventis
300 Somerset Corporate Blvd
Bridgewater, NJ 08807-2854
Telephone: (800) 981-2491
http://www.sanofi-aventis.us

Schering-Plough
Global Headquarters
2000 Galloping Hill Road
Kenilworth, NJ 07033-0530
Telephone: (908) 298-4000
http://www.schering-plough.com

Watson Pharmaceuticals
Corporate Headquarters
311 Bonnie Circle
Corona, CA 92880
Telephone: (951) 493-5300
http://www.watsonpharm.com

Wyeth
5 Giralda Farms
Madison, NJ 07940
Telephone: (973) 660-5500
http://www.wyeth.com

APPENDIX M

Common Sound-Alike Drug Names

The following is a list of common sound-alike drug names. Trade names are capitalized. In parentheses next to each drug name is the pharmacological classification/ use of the drug. (Reprinted from the *PDR Nurse's Drug Handbook* by G.R. Spratto and A.L. Woods. Clifton Park, NY: Thomson Delmar Learning, 2004.)

Accupril (ACE inhibitor)

acetazolamide (antiglaucoma drug)

Aciphex (proton pump inhibitor)

Aciphex (proton pump inhibitor)

Actos (oral hypoglycemic)

Adriamycin (antineoplastic)

albuterol (sympathomimetic)

Aldomet (antihypertensive)

Alkeran (antineoplastic)

Alkeran (antineoplastic)

allopurinol (antigout drug)

alprazolam (anti-anxiety agent)

Amaryl (oral hypoglycemic)

Accutane (anti-acne drug)

acetohexamide (oral antidiabetic drug)

Accupril (ACE inhibitor)

Aricept (anti-Alzheimer's drug)

Actonel (diphosphonate—bone-growth regulator)

Aredia (bone-growth regulator)

atenolol (beta-blocker)

Aldoril (antihypertensive)

Leukeran (antineoplastic)

Myleran (antineoplastic)

Apresoline (antihypertensive)

lorazepam (anti-anxiety agent)

Reminyl (anti-Alzheimer's drug)

Ambien (sedative-hypnotic)	Amen (progestin)
amiloride (diuretic)	amlodipine (calcium channel blocker)
amiodarone (anti-arrhythmic)	amrinone (inotropic agent)
amitriptyline (antidepressant)	nortriptyline (antidepressant)
Apresazide (antihypertensive)	Apresoline (antihypertensive)
Aripiprazole (antipsychotic)	Lansoprazole (proton pump inhibitor)
Arlidin (peripheral vasodilator)	Aralen (antimalarial)
Artane (cholinergic blocking agent)	Altace (ACE inhibitor)
Asacol (anti-inflammatory drug)	Avelox (fluoroquinolone antibiotic)
asparaginase (antineoplastic agent)	pegaspargase (antineoplastic agent)
Atarax (anti-anxiety agent)	Ativan (anti-anxiety agent)
atenolol (beta-blocker)	timolol (beta-blocker)
Atrovent (cholinergic blocking agent)	Alupent (sympathomimetic)

Avandia (oral hypoglycemic)	Coumadin (anticoagulant)
Avandia (oral hypoglycemic)	Prandin (oral hypoglycemic)
Bacitracin (antibacterial)	Bactroban (anti-infective, topical)
Benylin (expectorant)	Ventolin (sympathomimetic)
Brevital (barbiturate)	Brevibloc (beta-adrenergic blocker)
Bumex (diuretic)	Buprenex (narcotic analgesic)
bupropion (antidepressant; smoking deterrent)	buspirone (anti-anxiety agent)
Cafergot (analgesic)	Carafate (anti-ulcer drug)
calciferol (vitamin D)	calcitriol (vitamin D)
carboplatin (antineoplastic agent)	cisplatin (antineoplastic agent)
Cardene (calcium channel blocker)	Cardizem (calcium channel blocker)
Cardura (antihypertensive)	Ridaura (gold-containing anti-inflammatory)
Cataflam (NSAID)	Catapres (antihypertensive)

Catapres (antihypertensive)	Combipres (antihypertensive)
cefotaxime (cephalosporin)	cefoxitin (cephalosporin)
cefuroxime (cephalosporin)	deferoxamine (iron chelator)
Celebrex (NSAID)	Cerebyx (anticonvulsant)
Celebrex (NSAID)	Celera (antidepressant)
Cerebyx (anticonvulsant)	Celera (antidepressant)
chlorpromazine (antipsychotic)	chlorpropamide (oral antidiabetic)
chlorpromazine (antipsychotic)	prochlorperazine (antipsychotic)
chlorpromazine (antipsychotic)	promethazine (antihistamine)
Clinoril (NSAID)	Clozaril (antipsychotic)
clomipramine (antidepressant)	clomiphene (ovarian stimulant)
clonidine (antihypertensive)	Klonopin (anticonvulsant)
Combivir (AIDS drug combination)	Combivent (combination for COPD)

Cozaar (antihypertensive) — Zocor (antihyperlipidemic)

cyclobenzaprine (skeletal muscle relaxant) — cyproheptadine (antihistamine)

cyclophosphamide (antineoplastic) — cyclosporine (immunosuppressant)

cyclosporine (immunosuppressant) — cycloserine (antineoplastic)

Cytovene (antiviral drug) — Cytosar (antineoplastic)

Cytoxan (antineoplastic) — Cytotec (prostaglandin derivative)

Cytoxan (antineoplastic) — Cytosar (antineoplastic)

Dantrium (skeletal muscle relaxant) — danazol (gonadotropin inhibitor)

Darvocet-N (analgesic) — Darvon-N (analgesic)

daunorubicin (antineoplastic) — doxorubicin (antineoplastic)

desipramine (antidepressant) — diphenhydramine (antihistamine)

DiaBeta (oral hypoglycemic) — Zebeta (beta-adrenergic blocker)

digitoxin (cardiac glycoside) — digoxin (cardiac glycoside)

diphenhydramine (antihistamine)	dimenhydrinate (antihistamine)
dopamine (sympathomimetic)	dobutamine (sympathomimetic)
Edecrin (diuretic)	Eulexin (antineoplastic)
enalapril (ACE inhibitor)	Anafranil (antidepressant)
enalapril (ACE inhibitor)	Eldepryl (anti-Parkinson agent)
Eryc (erythromycin base)	Ery-Tab (erythromycin base)
etidronate (bone-growth regulator)	etretinate (antipsoriatic)
etomidate (general anesthetic)	etidronate (bone-growth regulator)
E-Vista (antihistamine)	Evista (estrogen receptor modulator)
Femara (antineoplastic)	Femhrt (estrogen-progestin combination)
Fioricet (analgesic)	Fiorinal (analgesic)
Flomax (alpha-adrenergic blocker)	Volmax (sympathomimetic)
flurbiprofen (NSAID)	fenoprofen (NSAID)

folinic acid (leucovorin calcium)   folic acid (vitamin B complex)

Gantrisin (sulfonamide)   Gantanol (sulfonamide)

glipizide (oral hypoglycemic)   glyburide (oral hypoglycemic)

glyburide (oral hypoglycemic)   Glucotrol (oral hypoglycemic)

Hycodan (cough preparation)   Hycomine (cough preparation)

hydralazine (antihypertensive)   hydroxyzine (anti-anxiety agent)

hydrocodone (narcotic analgesic)   hydrocortisone (corticosteroid)

Hydrogesic (analgesic combination)   hydroxyzine (antihistamine)

hydromorphone (narcotic analgesic)   morphine (narcotic analgesic)

Hydropres (antihypertensive)   Diupres (antihypertensive)

Hytone (topical corticosteroid)   Vytone (topical corticosteroid)

imipramine (antidepressant)   Norpramin (antidepressant)

Inderal (beta-adrenergic blocker)   Inderide (antihypertensive)

Inderal (beta-adrenergic blocker)	Isordil (coronary vasodilator)
Indocin (NSAID)	Minocin (antibiotic)
K-Phos Neutral (phosphorus-potassium replenishment)	Neutra-Phos-K (phosphorus-potassium replenishment)
Lamictal (anticonvulsant)	Lamisil (antifungal)
Lamictal (anticonvulsant)	Ludiomil (alpha- and beta-adrenergic blocker)
Lamisil (antiviral)	Ludiomil (alpha- and beta-adrenergic blocker)
Lanoxin (cardiac glycoside)	Lasix (diuretic)
Lantus (insulin glargine)	Lente insulin (insulin zinc suspension)
Lioresal (muscle relaxant)	lisinopril (ACE inhibitor)
Lithostat (lithium carbonate)	Lithobid (lithium carbonate)
Lithotabs (lithium carbonate)	Lithobid (lithium carbonate)
Lodine (NSAID)	codeine (narcotic analgesic)

Lopid (antihyperlipidemic)	Lorabid (beta-lactam antibiotic)
lovastatin (antihyperlipidemic)	Lotensin (ACE inhibitor)
Ludiomil (alpha- and beta- adrenergic blocker)	Lomotil (antidiarrheal)
Medrol (corticosteroid)	Haldol (antipsychotic)
metolazone (thiazide diuretic)	methotrexate (antineoplastic)
metolazone (thiazide diuretic)	metoclopramide (GI stimulant)
metoprolol tartrate (beta- adrenergic blocker)	metoclopramide hydrochloride (GI stimulant)
metoprolol (beta-adrenergic blocker)	misoprostol (prostaglandin derivative)
Monopril (ACE inhibitor)	minoxidil (antihypertensive)
nelfinavir (antiviral)	nevirapine (antiviral)
nicardipine (calcium channel blocker)	nifedipine (calcium channel blocker)
Norlutate (progestin)	Norlutin (progestin)
Noroxin (fluoroquinolone antibiotic)	Neurontin (anticonvulsant)

Norvasc (calcium channel blocker)	Navane (antipsychotic)
Norvir (antiviral)	Retrovir (antiviral)
Ocufen (NSAID)	Ocuflox (fluoroquinolone antibiotic)
Orinase (oral hypoglycemic)	Ornade (upper respiratory product)
Percocet (narcotic analgesic)	Percodan (narcotic analgesic)
paroxetine (antidepressant)	paclitaxel (antineoplastic)
Paxil (antidepressant)	paclitaxel (antineoplastic)
Paxil (antidepressant)	Taxol (antineoplastic)
penicillamine (heavy metal antagonist)	penicillin (antibiotic)
pindolol (beta-adrenergic blocker)	Parlodel (inhibitor of prolactin secretion)
Platinol (antineoplastic)	Paraplatin (antineoplastic)
Pletal (antiplatelet drug)	Plavix (antiplatelet drug)
Pravachol (antihyperlipidemic)	Prevacid (GI drug)

Pravachol (antihyperlipidemic)	propranolol (beta-adrenergic blocker)
prednisolone (corticosteroid)	prednisone (corticosteroid)
Prilosec (inhibitor of gastric acid secretion)	Prozac (antidepressant)
Prinivil (ACE inhibitor)	Prilosec (GI drug)
Prinivil (ACE inhibitor)	Proventil (sympathomimetic)
Procanbid (antiarrhythmic)	Procan SR (antiarrhythmic)
propranolol (beta-adrenergic blocker)	Propulsid (GI drug)
Provera (progestin)	Premarin (estrogen)
Prozac (antidepressant)	Proscar (androgen hormone inhibitor)
quinidine (anti-arrhythmic)	clonidine (antihypertensive)
quinidine (anti-arrhythmic)	Quinamm (antimalarial)
quinine (antimalarial)	quinidine (antiarrhythmic)
Regroton (antihypertensive)	Hygroton (diuretic)

APPENDIX N

Nomogram

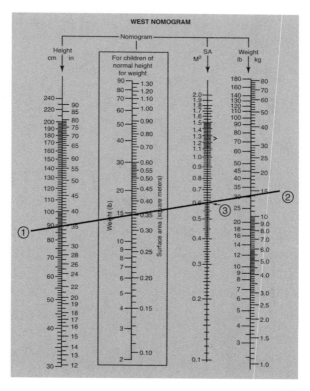

Drug Identification Guide

ACARBOSE
Precose
BAYER
Antidiabetic, oral; alpha-glucosidase inhibitor

25 mg   50 mg   100 mg

ACETAMINOPHEN AND HYDROCODONE BITARTRATE
Vicodin
ABBOTT
Analgesic

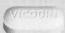

500 mg / 5 mg

Vicodin ES
ABBOTT

7.5 mg / 750 mg

Vicodin HP
ABBOTT

10 mg / 660 mg

ACETAMINOPHEN AND OXYCODONE HCl
Percocet
ENDO
Analgesic

325 mg / 2.5 mg

325 mg / 5 mg

325 mg / 7.5 mg

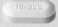

325 mg / 10 mg

500 mg / 7.5 mg

650 mg / 10 mg

ALENDRONATE SODIUM
Fosamax
MERCK
Bone growth regulator, biphosphonate

5 mg

10 mg   35 mg

 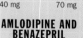

40 mg   70 mg

AMLODIPINE AND BENAZEPRIL
Lotrel
NOVARTIS
Calcium channel blocker

2.5 mg

5 mg

10 mg

AMPHETAMINE MIXTURES

Adderall XR
SHIRE

CNS stimulant

5 mg

ATENOLOL

Tenormin
ASTRAZENECA

Beta-adrenergic blocking agent

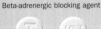

ATOMOXETINE HCI

Strattera
ELI LILLY

Antidepressant, selective
serotonin reuptake inhibitor

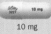

10 mg

18 mg

25 mg

40 mg

60 mg

BENAZEPRIL HCI

Lotensin
NOVARTIS

Antihypertensive, ACE inhibitor

5 mg   10 mg

20 mg   40 mg

Lotensin HCT
NOVARTIS

5 mg

Lotensin HCT
NOVARTIS

10 mg

Lotensin HCT
NOVARTIS

20 mg

BUDESONIDE

Pulmicort Respules
ASTRAZENECA

Glucocorticoid

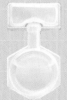

CANDESARTAN CILEXETIL

Atacand
ASTRAZENECA LP

Antihypertensive, angiotensin II
receptor blocker

CAPECITABINE

Xeloda
LA ROCHE

Antineoplastic, antimetabolite

150 mg

500 mg

CARBAMAZEPINE

Tegretol
NOVARTIS

Anticonvulsant

100 mg   200 mg

CEPHALEXIN HCI MONOHYDRATE

Keflex
ADVANCIS

Cephalosporin, first generation

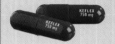

750 mg

CIPROFLOXACIN HCI

Cipro
BAYER

Antibiotic, fluoroquinolone

100 mg   250 mg

500 mg

750 mg

Cipro XR
BAYER

500 mg

Cipro XR
BAYER

1000 mg

CLARITHROMYCIN
Biaxin
ABBOTT
Antibiotic, macrolide

250 mg

500 mg

Biaxin XL
ABBOTT

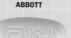

500 mg

CLONAZEPAM
Klonopin
LA ROCHE
Anticonvulsant

0.5 mg

1 mg

2 mg

CYCLOBENZAPRINE HCI
Flexeril
MERCK
Skeletal muscle relaxant,
centrally acting

DEXMETHYLPHENIDATE
HCI
Focalin
NOVARTIS
CNS stimulant

2.5 mg

5 mg

10 mg

DIAZEPAM
Valium
LA ROCHE
Antianxiety, benzodiazepine

2 mg

5 mg

10 mg

DICLOFENAC SODIUM
Voltaren
NOVARTIS
Non steroidal anti-inflammatory

25 mg

50 mg

75 mg

ESOMEPRAZOLE MG
Nexium
ASTRAZENECA
Proton pump inhibitor

20 mg

EZETIMIBE
Zetia
MERCK
Antihyperlipidemic, HMG-CoA
reductase inhibitor

FELODIPINE
Plendil
ASTRAZENECA
Calcium channel blocker

FENOFIBRATE
Tricor
ABBOTT
Antihyperlipidemic

48 mg

145 mg

FINASTERIDE
Proscar
ABBOTT
Androgen hormone inhibitor

5 mg

FLUOXETINE HCl
Prozac
ELI-LILLY
Antidepressant, selective serotonin reuptake inhibitor

10 mg

20 mg

FLUVASTATIN SODIUM
Lescol
NOVARTIS
Antihyperlipidemic, HMG-CoA reductase inhibitor

20 mg

40 mg

GRANISETRON HCl
Kytril
LA ROCHE
Antiemetic, 5-HT3 receptor antagonist

1 mg

HYDROCODONE BITARTRATE/ HOMATROPINE METHYBROMIDE
Hycodan
ENDO
Analgesic

KETOROLAC TROMETHAMINE
Toradol oral
LA ROCHE
Nonsteroidal anti-inflammatoryn

10 mg

LEVOTHYROXINE SODIUM (T4)
Levoxyl
KING
Thyroid product

23 mg   50 mg

75 mg   88 mg

100 mg   112 mg

125 mg   137 mg

150 mg   175 mg

200 mg   300 mg

LEVOTHYROXINE SODIUM (T4)
Synthroid
ABBOTT
Thyroid product

LISINOPRIL
Prinivil
MERCK
Antihypertensive, ACE inhibitor

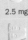

2.5 mg

5 mg

10 mg

20 mg

40 mg

LISINOPRIL
Zestril
ASTRAZENECA
Antihypertensive, ACE inhibitor

LOPINAVIR/RITONAVIR
Kaletra
ABBOTT
HIV protease inhibitor

LOSARTAN HCTZ
Hyzaar
MERCK
Angiotensin II receptor antagonist and diuretic

LOSARTAN POTASSIUM
Cozaar
MERCK

Antihypertensive, angiotensin II
receptor blocker

25 mg

50 mg

100 mg

LOVASTATIN
Mevacor
MERCK

Antihyperlipidemic, HMG-CoA
reductase inhibitor

10 mg

20 mg

40 mg

METAXALONE
Skelaxin
KING

Muscle relaxant

METFORMIN
Fortamet
FIRST HORIZON

Antidiabetic, oral; biguanide

METHYLPHENIDATE HCl
Ritalin
NOVARTIS

CNS stimulant

5 mg

10 mg

20 mg

METOPROLOL SUCCINATE
Toprol
ASTRAZENECA

Beta-adrenergic blocking agent

METOPROLOL TARTRATE
Lopressor
NOVARTIS

Beta-adrenergic blocking agent

25/100 mg

50/100 mg

50 mg

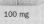

100 mg

MONTELUKAST SODIUM
Singulair
MERCK

Antiasthmatic, leukotriene
receptor antagonist

MOXIFLOXACIN HCl
Avelox
BAYER

Antibiotic, fluoroquinolone

NAPROXEN
Naprosyn
LA ROCHE

Nonsteroidal anti-inflammatory

NAPROXEN SODIUM
Anaprox
LA ROCHE

Nonsteroidal anti-inflammatory

NITROFURANTOIN
Macrobid
PROCTOR AND GAMBLE
Antibiotic

NITROFURANTOIN
Macrodantin
PROCTOR AND GAMBLE
Antibiotic

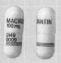

OLANZAPINE
Zyprexa
ELI LILLY
Antipsychotic

2.5 mg

5 mg

7.5 mg

10 mg

15 mg

20 mg

Zyprexa Zydia
ELI LILLY

15 mg

Zyprexa Zydia
ELI LILLY

20 mg

OSELTAMIVIR PHOSPHATE
Tamiflu
LA ROCHE
Antiviral

QUETIAPINE FUMARATE
Seroquel
ASTRAZENECA
Antipsychotic

OXYCODONE AND ACETAMINOPHEN
Endocet
ENDO
Analgesic

5 mg / 325 mg

7.5 mg / 325 mg

10 mg / 325 mg

7.5 mg / 500 mg

10 mg / 650 mg

POTASSIUM SALTS
Klor-con and Klor-con M20
UPSHER SMITH
Electrolyte

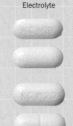

RALOXIFENE HCl
Evista
ELI LILLY
Estrogen receptor modulator

RISEDRONATE SODIUM
Actonel
PROCTOR AND GAMBLE

Bone growth regulator, biphosphonate

5 mg

30 mg

35 mg

RIVASTIGMINE TARTRATE
Exelon
NOVARTIS

Treatment of Alzheimer's Disease

1 mg

3 mg

4.5 mg

6 mg

RIZATRIPTAN BENZOATE
Maxalt
MERCK

5 mg

10 mg

Maxalt MLT
MERCK

5 mg

Maxalt MLT
MERCK
Antimigraine

10 mg

ROFECOXIB
Vioxx
MERCK

Nonsteroidal anti-inflammatory; COX-2 inhibitor

ROSUVASTATIN
Crestor
ASTRAZENECA

Antihyperlipidemic, HMG-CoA reductase inhibitor

SIMVASTATIN
Zocor
MERCK

Antihyperlipidemic, HMG-CoA reductase inhibitor

5 mg

10 mg

20 mg

40 mg

80 mg

SPIRONOLACTONE
Aldactone
MYLAN

Diuretic, potassium-sparing

TAMOXIFEN CITRATE

Nolvadex
ASTRAZENECA
Antiestrogen

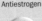
22.5 mg

30 mg

ZAFIRLUKAST

Accolate
ASTRAZENECA
Antiasthmatic

TEGASEROD MALEATE

Zelnorm
NOVARTIS

Drug for irritable bowel
syndrome in women

5 mg   6 mg

TRIAMTERENE AND HYDROCHLOROTHIAZIDE

Maxide
MYLAN

Antihypertensive,
combination drug

ZOLMITRIPTAN

Zomig
ASTRAZENECA
Antimigraine

TEMAZEPAM

Restoril
MALLINCKRODT

Sedative-hypnotic,
benzodiazepine

7.5 mg

15 mg

VALGANCICLOVIR HCl

Valcyte
LA ROCHE

Antiviral

20 mg

Glossary

additive effect—Effect wherein two or more substances used in combination produce a total effect that is the same as the sum of the individual effects.

antagonism—What happens when two drugs act to decrease the effects of each other.

antidote—A drug or substance given to stop a toxic effect.

antineoplastic agents—Drugs used to treat cancers and malignant neoplasms.

bar coding—Placing a code on packaging to help standardize and regulate inventory control.

beaker—A device in which materials to be heated are placed.

birthday rule—Determines the primary payer when the patient is a child living with both parents and each parent carries health insurance. The parent with the earlier birthday in the calendar year is the primary insurer for the child.

brand name—A word, symbol, or device assigned to a product by its manufacturer, registered or not registered, as a trademark of its identity.

calibration—The number of drops that equal 1 milliliter for a particular type of IV tubing; also called the drop factor.

capsule—A solid dosage form in which the drug is enclosed in either a hard or soft shell of soluble material.

Centers for Medicare & Medicaid (CMS)—An organization that inspects and approves institutions to provide Medicaid and Medicare services.

central IV line—An intravenous line that enters the body through a large vein in the neck or chest.

certified pharmacy technician (CPhT)—A person who has passed the Pharmacy Technician Certification Examination (PTCE) developed and administered by the Pharmacy Technician Certification Board (PTCB).

CHAMPVA—Civilian Health and Medical Program of the Veterans Administration; a program to cover medical expenses of the dependent spouse and children of veterans with total, permanent service-connected disabilities.

chemical name—Drug name derived from the chemical composition of the drug.

child-resistant containers—Packaging designed to be difficult for children under the age of five to access.

class A prescription balance—A two-pan device that may be used for weighing small amounts of drugs (not more than 120 g).

clean claim—An error-free insurance claim.

coinsurance—The amount or percentage the insured is responsible for after the deductible has been met.

community pharmacy—Provides pharmaceutical services to the general public; also known as retail pharmacy.

complex fraction—The numerator or the denominator or both as a whole number, proper fraction, or mixed number. The value may be less than, greater than, or equal to 1.

compounding slab—A plate made of ground glass with a hard, flat, and nonabsorbent surface for mixing compounds.

continuous—Related to an infusion of an intravenous drug administered steadily over a period of time.

controlled substance—Drug that has a potential for abuse and which leads to physical or psychological dependence.

convulsion—Abnormal motor movements.

co-pay, co-payment—Amount of money the patient owes at each visit; this varies with insurers from $5 to $25, or more.

counter balance—A device capable of weighing much larger quantities, up to about 5 kg. It is a double-pan balance.

CPT codes—Common Procedural Terminology, a coding system used to describe services and procedures.

database applications—Electronic storage of information for retrieval, searching, and reprocessing of information.

DEA Form 41—Form used to report disposal of a controlled substance.

DEA Form 106—Form used to report the significant loss of controlled substances.

DEA Form 222—Form used to acquire schedule II substances from a supplier.

deductible—A specific amount of money that must be paid each year before the policy benefits begin (for example, $50, $100, $300, or $500).

demulcence—An agent that soothes inflamed or irritated tissues.

denominator—The number the whole is divided into.

Department of Public Health (DPH)—An organization that oversees hospitals, including the pharmacy department.

depression—An agent that decreases some body function or activity.

digits—symbols used in the Arabic number system (1, 2, 3, 4, 5, 6, 7, 8, 9, 10); also known as integers.

displacement—The transfer of impulses from one expression to another, such as from fighting to talking.

drop factor—The number of drops that equal 1 milliliter for a particular type of IV tubing; also called the calibration.

dropper bottle—Container used for dispensing ophthalmic, nasal, otic, or oral liquids to be administered by drops.

drug action—The physiological change in the body or the response to the drug effect.

drug interaction—An interference of a drug with the effect of another drug, nutrient, or laboratory test.

drug recall—Removal of defective, ineffective, or unsafe drug products from the marketplace.

enteric-coated tablet—A tablet covered in a special coating to protect it from stomach acid, allowing the drug to dissolve in the intestines.

explanation of benefits (EOB)—Document sent from the insurance company to the patient outlining payments made for services and patient responsibilities.

extremes—The two outside terms in a ratio.

floor stock system—A system of drug distribution in which drugs are issued in bulk form and stored in medication rooms on patient care units.

generic name—The name the manufacturer uses for a drug.

graduate—A device used to measure liquids.

group health plan—A plan arranged by an employer or special interest group for the benefit of members and their dependents.

group purchasing—Procurement contracts are negotiated on behalf of the members of a group (for example, hospitals, nursing home pharmacies, and home infusion pharmacies). The group-purchasing organization uses the collective buying power of its members to negotiate discounts from manufacturers, wholesalers, and other suppliers.

Hazard Communication Standard (HCS)—An OSHA standard intended to increase health-care practitioners' awareness of risks, improve work practices and appropriate use of personal protective equipment, and reduce injuries and illnesses in the workplace.

HCPCS codes—The Health Care Finance Administration Common Procedure Coding System uses a set of standardized numbers to denote billable medical devices.

Health Insurance Portability and Accountability Act (HIPAA)—Legislation enacted to project patient privacy in the electronic transfer of data.

Health Maintenance Organization (HMO)—Organization that provides services to covered persons in an individual, group, or public health plan.

heat gun—An instrument used for melting and polishing.

hot plate—A heated iron plate used to heat substances (usually adjustable between 50 and 300 degrees Celsius) as may be required for compounding.

ICD-9-CM codes—The International Classification of Diseases 9th Revision is a set of standardized numbers used to denote diseases.

improper fraction—The numerator is greater than or equal to the denominator.

independent purchasing—The director of the pharmacy or buyer directly contacts and negotiates pricing with pharmaceutical manufacturers.

individual health plan—A plan issued to one person.

induction—The period of time between the beginning of administration of a general anesthetic and the point at which the patient has achieved the desired level of unconsciousness.

inhibition—The arrest of a process normally performed by a molecule of a drug.

inscription—Name of the drug, amount, and concentration prescribed.

insurance premium—The amount of money paid by a policy holder to an insurance company for coverage.

integers—Symbols used in the Arabic number system (1, 2, 3, 4, 5, 6, 7, 8, 9, 10); also known as digits.

intermittent—Related to an infusion of an intravenous drug administered at specific intervals or time periods.

intravenous route—Route used when it is necessary for medication to enter the blood circulation directly.

inventory—The stock of medications a pharmacy keeps immediately on hand.

inventory turnover rate—A mathematical calculation used to determine the number of times the average inventory is replaced over a period of time, usually annually.

invoice—A form describing a purchase and the amount due.

irritation—An agent that causes inflammation of tissues.

Joint Commission—An organization that surveys and accredits health-care organizations.

legend drug—A medication that may be dispensed only with a prescription; also known as a prescription drug.

mail-order pharmacy—A licensed pharmacy that uses the mail or other carriers (for example, overnight carriers or parcel services) to deliver prescriptions to patients.

markup—The difference between the cost of merchandise and its selling price.

means—The two inside terms in a ratio.

Medicaid—A federal/state medical assistance program to provide health insurance for specific populations.

Medicare—A federal health insurance program created as part of the Social Security Act.

medication order—The written order for particular medications and services to be provided to a patient within an institutional setting; medication orders are written by physicians, nurse practitioners, or physician's assistants.

mixed number—A whole number and a proper fraction that are combined. The value of the mixed number is always greater than 1.

mortar—A cup-shaped vessel in which materials are ground or crushed.

National Drug Code (NDC)—A unique and permanent product code assigned to each new drug as it becomes available in the marketplace; it identifies the manufacturer or distributor, the drug formulation, and the size and type of its packaging.

Occupational Safety and Health Administration (OSHA)—A regulating body concerned with writing and enforcing standards for health and safety in the workplace.

ointment jar—Container used to dispense semisolid dosage forms such as creams and ointments.

over-the-counter (OTC)—A medication that may be purchased without a prescription directly from the pharmacy.

package inserts—Information about the drug that is disseminated to patients on packaging or special inserts that accompany the dispensed drug.

Parkinson's disease—A disorder characterized by resting tremor, rigidity or resistance to passive movement, akinesia, and loss of postural reflexes.

percent—A fraction whose numerator is expressed and whose denominator is understood to be 100.

peripheral IV line—An intravenous line that enters the body through the veins of the arm.

pestle—A solid device that is used to crush or grind materials in a mortar.

Physician's Order Sheet—A medication order for inpatients written by physicians.

pipette—A long, thin, calibrated hollow tube, which is made of glass used for measuring liquids.

potentiation—One drug prolongs the effects of another drug.

preauthorization—The requirement of notification and permission to receive additional types of services before one obtains those services.

preferred providers—physicians and pharmacists who contract with insurance carriers to provide patient care at a discounted rate.

preferred provider organization (PPO)—A managed care organization that contracts with a group of providers, who are called *preferred providers,* to offer services to the managed care organization's members.

prepaid health-care program—A plan whereby services are rendered by physicians or facilities who elect to participate in a user program for services.

prescription—An order for medication issued by a physician, dentist, or other properly licensed medical provider.

prescription bottle—Container used for dispensing liquids of low viscosity.

primary IV line—The main route of the drug entering into the circulatory system.

proper fraction—The numerator is smaller than the denominator and designates less than one whole unit.

proprietary drugs—Drugs created and distributed by a particular manufacturer. The proprietary name is the trade or brand name of the drug.

quality assurance—The adjustment of quality-control procedures and systems as needed.

quality control—An organized effort of all individuals directly or indirectly involved in the production, packaging, and distribution of quality medications, which are safe, effective, and acceptable.

receptor—The cell to which a drug has an affinity.

retail pharmacy—Provides pharmaceutical services to the general public; also known as community pharmacy.

right-to-know laws—Regulations enacted by states that allow employees access to information about their duties, rights, responsibilities, and on-the-job hazards.

secondary IV line—An additional route of the drug entering the body through the veins by adding the medication to an already existing primary IV line.

signature—Relates to the part of the prescription that provides patient instructions; also called the transcription.

solution—A liquid dosage form in which active ingredients are dissolved in a liquid vehicle.

State Board of Pharmacy (BOP)—An agency that registers pharmacists and pharmacy technicians.

stimulation—Caused by an agent that increases the activity of a cell, tissue, organ, or the whole body.

subscription—Dispensing directions to a pharmacist.

summation—Combining drugs to achieve the expected effect of each drug.

suppository—A small, solid body shaped for ready introduction into one of the orifices of the body other than the oral cavity (for example, rectum, urethra, or vagina), made of a substance, usually medicated, that is solid at ordinary temperature but melts at body temperature.

suspension—A liquid dosage form that contains solid drug particles floating in a liquid medium.

symbol—Numbers used by the Roman numeral system, for example, I, V, and X. The system uses seven basic symbols and various combinations of these symbols to represent all numbers in the Arabic number system. Roman numerals can be written as uppercase or lowercase letters.

synergism—The cooperative effect of two or more drugs given together to produce a stronger effect than that of either drug given alone.

third-party payer—The fee for services provided is paid by an insurance company and not by the patient.

tongs—Devices used for handling hot beakers.

trade name—A drug name, followed by the symbol ®, which indicates that the name is registered to a specific manufacturer or owner and that no one else can use it.

transcription—Relates to the part of the prescription that provides patient instructions; also called the signature.

TRICARE—A federally funded comprehensive health benefits program for dependents of personnel serving in the uniformed services.

turnover—The rate at which inventory is used or the number of days it takes for the stock of an item to be used.

vehicle—In pharmacy, the substance added to a drug to give the drug bulk or suitable consistency.

venipuncture—The intentional piercing of a vein for any purpose, such as withdrawal of blood for a laboratory test.

vial—A small glass or plastic bottle intended to hold medicine.

want book—A list of drugs and devices that routinely need to be reordered.

Index